THE BOOK OF
PAIN RELIEF

BY THE SAME AUTHOR

Acupuncture Treatment of Pain
Candida Albicans
Chelation Therapy
Clear Body, Clear Mind
Natural Life Extension
Osteopathic Self Treatment
Palpatory Literacy
Probiotics (with Natasha Trenev)
Soft Tissue Manipulation
The Stress Protection Plan
Thorsons Guide to Amino Acids

THE BOOK OF
PAIN RELIEF

Leon Chaitow
DO, MRO, ND

Thorsons
An Imprint of HarperCollinsPublishers

For Carol and Irwin with love.

Thorsons
An Imprint of HarperCollins*Publishers*
77–85 Fulham Palace Road,
Hammersmith, London W6 8JB

First published by Thorsons 1993

1 3 5 7 9 10 8 6 4 2

A catalogue record for this book
is available from the British Library

ISBN 0 7225 2820 5

Typeset by Harper Phototypesetters Limited,
Northampton, England
Printed in Great Britain by
Woolnough Bookbinding, Irthlingborough, Northamptonshire

Contents

The puzzle of pain

Acute pain (short and sharp) is often a danger warning which, if ignored, can lead to injury, and it may also be a reminder that you have been overdoing things, and that you need to rest and recover. In this capacity acute pain is usually useful – even vital – as a protective mechanism. On the other hand, chronic pain (long continued) does not seem to offer any clear advantage and is very often, and in most senses of the word, 'useless'.

It would, however, be wrong to try to deal with chronic pain without understanding its cause, even though it may not be possible to remove the cause. Having established this, attention can be focused on the pain itself in an effort to modify, reduce, calm or ease it. Left untreated chronic pain can rapidly trigger physical and emotional problems.

About one person in every three suffers from some degree of chronic pain, and one in five will be partially or totally disabled by this during some period of their lives – statistics which have made the artificial removal of pain by medication an enormous industry. Fortunately, though, non-drug methods of pain relief are also available, and some come from inside our bodies.

NATURAL PAIN KILLERS WITHIN

A cut heals and a broken bone mends without outside help (other than the obvious first-aid measures), so we should not be too surprised to find that a provision has also been made within our bodies for the easing of pain. This is by the production of endorphins and enkephalins (opiate-like pain-killing substances produced by the brain), as well as by alterations in our psychological behaviour. Many of the self-help methods used against pain, as well as treatments given to reduce its intensity, depend for their success on the release of these natural substances and on altering the way pain is transmitted to the brain.

MANY TREATMENT CHOICES

When additional help is needed we are fortunate that variety is not lacking in the ways of treating and self-treating pain. We are almost spoiled for choice with a confusing array of chemical (medication by drugs, herbs or homoeopathic remedies), physical, electrical, electromagnetic and psychological means, as well as some extraordinary and apparently esoteric methods, all claiming success rates and asking to be tried.

The choice of the method or methods most likely to be helpful and effective in a particular case is best left to qualified practitioners, but sadly many are trained to use only one or at most a couple of systems and means of pain control, and they may be ignorant of, or prejudiced against, other methods. This is why specialist pain clinics which offer a wide range of approaches and techniques, performed by a variety of therapists, are the ideal places to look for help if you are suffering from chronic pain.

No single method or combination of methods can be said to always work, and often any of several choices can be equally successful, so trial and error is sometimes the only way to discover what is best.

PHYSICAL OR MENTAL?

Many experts believe that the nature of pain can best be understood by looking at its physical side – concentrating on the nervous system – while others emphasize the importance of its emotional and psychological characteristics. The truth is that both physical and psychological elements are usually intimately combined in most cases of chronic pain, and *both* usually require attention when dealing with long-term pain.

The experience of many thousands of therapists and researchers is that when a person suffering pain understands the causes, nature, mechanism and role of pain, a vital step has been taken in the successful handling of the problem. An added bonus comes if, as well as understanding it, the sufferer can acquire at least some ability to control aspects of the pain.

For example, there are many forms of headache which can be successfully treated by:

- medication (herbal such as with feverfew; or by use of an appropriate drug)
- acupuncture (which has a high success rate)
- osteopathic or chiropractic treatment of the neck and head
- relaxation exercises or use of biofeedback
- alterations of diet if allergy, sensitivity or toxicity were the cause of the headache
- postural re-education if habits of posture prove to be the underlying cause

So, which of these is the correct treatment? The ones which deal with both cause and symptom would be first choice, but, if no cause could be found, the one(s) which did the least harm in terms of side-effects, and which allowed the sufferer some degree of control over symptoms, would be best.

UNDERSTANDING AND CONTROL

Both understanding and control are extremely important in helping to deal with chronic pain. The opinion of many experts is that there is almost certainly a need for a combination of both psychological (coming to terms with it; learning to control aspects of it; understanding it) and physical elements (in their broadest sense, including the use of anything from medication to acupuncture or manipulative strategies) in the successful handling of most chronic and stubborn pain problems.

CONTROL = EMPOWERMENT = SELF-HELP

Central to what is done to and for a person in pain is the need for that person to start to take some degree of control of the situation, to feel empowered to influence the processes at work and not to feel themselves to be a mere object, simply the helpless recipient of other people's efforts. *Self-help* measures are therefore very important in this process, although they should not just be picked randomly but rather as part of a total approach to sufferers and their problems.

This means that any self-help method should work together with whatever help is being offered professionally. This is true whether self-help involves learning to use simple hydrotherapy measures – such as hot and cold compresses, or ice massage – or performing special stretching exercises, doing deep relaxation exercises, using electrical pain relieving machines such as TENS (transcutaneous electrical nerve stimulation), or anything else which helps to modify pain and *which does no harm*.

SHORT-TERM (ACUTE) AND LONG-TERM (CHRONIC) PAIN

Fortunately for us, pain usually lasts only a short time, leaving nothing but a memory of its presence. Even more fortunately we don't retain an actual 'recording' of the intensity of the pain we have experienced. However, the memory that it happened can help us not to do certain things again, or to do them more carefully next time.

An army of people, though, can testify to the fact that pain is not always merely a short-lived and useful warning, and in order to deal effectively with that sort of pain we need to know more about some of its unusual and sometimes confusing features.

SOCIAL VARIATIONS

While the mechanisms by which pain is felt may be the same in all people, and while it is registered via the nervous system and brain in the same way by all people, its reported intensity (how it is perceived) differs from person to person, depending upon social and cultural factors. For example, a person from northern Europe and a person from the Mediterranean area, both exposed to identical pain (say a pin prick on the arm) will report what they feel quite differently although the way their respective nervous systems deal with the pin-prick is identical. One will complain of 'discomfort' and the other of 'great pain'. Why should this be? It is thought that it is because of social differences, since the way pain is perceived, seen, reported and handled has a lot to do with our upbringing and culture.

DIFFERENT SITUATIONS, DIFFERENT PAIN?

The very same injury or source of pain, no matter how intense, will be felt differently (to a very large extent) under different circumstances. For example, someone may receive a violent injury during intense activity, such as in battle or during a sporting event, and feel no pain until after the emotionally and mentally supercharged activity is over, when the pain will usually become all too apparent.

Two of the main researchers into pain, Drs Melzack and Wall, have shown that more than one in three people arriving at emergency clinics with severe injuries, including large lacerations, amputated fingers and bone fractures, reported feeling little or no pain until many hours after the injury. They report that 65 per cent of soldiers seriously injured in battle, and one in five of the public undergoing major operations, report feeling almost no pain afterwards, sometimes for days.

On the other hand, excruciating pains are sometimes reported in which no cause can be discovered, something frequently seen in cases of acute low back problems.

The reason for these extremes (no pain with obvious injury and great pain without much injury) is not yet understood, but as researchers make clear – it is now known that there are biological mechanisms that set a limit on pain. What we *think* about the pain, how afraid or anxious we are about it, what we believe it represents in health terms, all influence how much pain we report. The same abdominal pain/discomfort may just seem a nuisance when it is thought to be the result of indigestion, but it would not be shrugged off so lightly were it thought that it might be because of a cancer or other serious condition.

The aches and pains following exercise are accepted because we know that they will vanish in a day or so, while the same discomfort caused by a wasting disease or an arthritic condition might be complained of as unbearable and in urgent need of help. Pain becomes a greater or lesser problem depending on what we think about it.

PAIN WHICH HELPS

Pain can sometimes be extremely useful, indeed life-saving, as shown by the disastrous lives of people born with a defect which prevents them from feeling pain. Self-inflicted yet unintentional injuries such as biting off bits of the tongue, as well as burns and breaks which are sustained without awareness of pain almost always result in a very short and unhappy life for such rare individuals.

We can surely all remember pain which stopped us from being burned when handling something hot. Here we see the opposite of the situation in which no pain is felt until some time after an injury – in fact we feel strong pain even before the injury has happened. So we learn not to repeat certain actions (touching a fire) and few would doubt the value to our lives of such short and sharp lessons. Not all pain has such value.

PAIN WHICH HAS NO PURPOSE

In many chronic conditions pain has long since served its useful purpose as a 'warning', and remains as nothing but a nuisance.

Take as an example the phantom pain frequently felt by amputees in their no-longer present limbs, or of pain which persists long after an injured area has healed. This type of 'useless' pain forms a major part of the problem of pain, involving enormous costs in terms of medication and therapy, as well as causing a vast degree of misery and disability.

PAIN OUT OF PROPORTION TO ITS CAUSE

Sometimes pain which is felt and accurately reported is out of all proportion to its apparent cause. This happens when someone is passing a kidney stone. As this passes down the ureter there is only minor mechanical irritation as well as a small amount of muscular pressure resulting from back-pressure of urine which cannot pass through it, and yet this produces agonizing pain (said to be among the most awful of pains).

This contrast between the cause and degree of pain is even harder to understand largely because the nerve supply to the ureter is so slight. The mystery becomes even greater when you consider the instant relief felt once the stone has passed.

Sometimes great levels of pain may be acting to prevent movement, assisting recovery through rest, and in such a case pain could be said to have some survival value.

PAIN WHICH RESULTS FROM SELF-PERPETUATING 'FACILITATED' AREAS

Because of mechanical and other forms of stress certain areas of the body, either alongside the spine, or in easily stressed parts of muscles (or near scars or old injuries) can become 'facilitated'. This means that the nervous impulses which pass through, or which actually derive from them, become extremely sensitive, easily activated, and capable of causing quite severe pain in distant 'target' areas. These rogue areas are called trigger points and they are a source of so much pain that they deserve special attention.

Such trigger points and focal points can be treated successfully, using either pain-killing injections, acupuncture, acupressure, soft-tissue manipulation techniques, electrotherapy or other methods, all of which will be explained in this book.

LESSONS AND MYSTERIES

These examples show something of the mystery and the importance of pain. How it acts to teach us, to warn us, to immobilize us . . . at times all-protective and useful in terms of survival. We also see that at other times pain has no obvious benefit, that it is all too often nothing but a relic of the past or even an aberration, and that we need to be able to find ways of reducing its potentially crippling influence on normal life. When pain is acting as an alarm, to warn and protect us, it would be foolish to kill the pain and ignore the message – for example, taking pain-killers when you have severe abdominal pain (possibly appendicitis) would be madness. Just suppressing such pain could lead to disaster.

On the other hand, if an alarm goes off and there is no underlying cause for it, or if the cause is long past, then no useful purpose is being served by the alarm being allowed to continue ringing! The trick is to know which pain is worth taking notice of as a warning and which should be got rid of as a nuisance.

WHERE DO WE FEEL PAIN?

Pain is felt in the brain, which receives a vast number of messages each second from 'reporting stations' sited throughout the body. The reporting stations are minute neural structures which send a host of different sorts of information (not just pain) back to the central nervous system, up the spinal cord, to different parts of the brain. The sorts of messages which are sent in an almost constant stream include information from every part of the body regarding warmth, cold, internal temperature, pressure, degree of stretch in tissues, light touch, changes in position as well as rate of change in position, and so on.

Those very special neural receptors which pass pain messages are called nociceptors and consist of free nerve endings which are literally receivers and transmitters of pain sensations. Some neural reporting stations pass messages only when strongly stimulated while others pass messages when very lightly stimulated, and some pass them along swift channels of communication (fast fibres) while others pass them along more leisurely channels (slow fibres).

In sorting out how pain works researchers have had to make sense of the ways in which the brain sorts out its priorities, faced as it is with this flood of continuous information coming from every part of the body all at once. Early theories seemed to suggest that by tracing the pathways along which pain messages were passing, and by interrupting these, by surgery if necessary, severe chronic pain could be stopped. This has been found not to be the case.

When spinal cord pathways are surgically cut in such attempts there are many failures, and sometimes matters are made worse, with new pains and even an exaggeration of old ones. We still have much to learn about pain! Pain is felt in the brain, physically, biochemically and neurologically. But that only tells us *how* the brain gets messages, and *how* these get through and are recorded. *What* we feel is something else altogether.

WHAT DECIDES WHAT WE FEEL?

Because physical methods of treatment are not universally successful in dealing with serious and chronic pain (although in many cases they are) we need also to turn to the way the mind, rather than the brain alone, handles the experience of pain. We need to look at how we ourselves remember, understand, think of and consider pain.

If we have learned, usually from childhood, to be alarmed at the presence of pain, to fear it, to be anxious about it (and society and commercial interests selling pain-killers reinforce this common response to pain), we are likely to 'feel' far more pain and discomfort than someone who has learned from childhood to observe pain, to try to understand it and act accordingly, not to fear it, not to become anxious about it, to behave as though it were just one more sensation such as tiredness, or hunger or pleasure.

Pain is a personal experience and we bring to it and to our handling of it all that we have learned and experienced in the past, all that has been said to us about it culturally and in our upbringing, all that we have observed and absorbed in our lives up to now in relation to health, disease and pain, and their implications.

Ask yourself:

- Do you see pain as something very important, deserving and demanding great attention, needing to be explained and the sooner the better?
- Do you see pain as calling out for relief, whatever the cause, as a first priority?

- Do you let the world know you are in pain, as loudly and often as you feel is your right?
- Do you hold back expression of the pain, keeping it to yourself, as it is no-one's business but your own, and anyway showing your feelings is not done?
- Do you secretly, deep down, see your pain as a means of gaining attention, as it used to when you were very young?
- Are you a stoic or a cry-baby?

DON'T JUDGE THE WAY YOU HANDLE PAIN!

Cultural factors over which you had no control influence the answers you gave to these questions, so don't be judgemental in any way whatsoever. One way of personally dealing with pain is not 'good' and another 'bad', since both are correct and proper for different cultures. The differences do, however, influence the degree of pain perceived, and while one way of dealing with pain might well seem more life enhancing or less stress inducing than another, this is open to debate.

Pain is therefore a remarkable combination of a physical phenomenon and an interpretation which our unique experiences and learning history bring to it. Dealing successfully with chronic pain demands that all parts of this combination be understood. Not just the physical, not just the emotional/psychological, but both.

This book explains many ways of handling pain, acute and chronic, and you will learn about:

- medical methods of treatment
- simple nutritional strategies which can influence pain levels
- musculoskeletal methods of treatment (including treating trigger points)
- hydrotherapy approaches
- traditional homoeopathic, herbal (and aromatherapy) methods
- The use of counter-irritation through acupuncture and acupressure
- Transcutaneous Electrical Nerve Stimulation (TENS) units and their safe home use
- the amazing use of healing/Therapeutic Touch

- stress reduction methods (including yoga breathing, meditation, relaxation and visualization)
- biofeedback machines in self-treatment
- psychological strategies and hypnosis methods
- the power of placebo in pain control and how this can be used

There are also special sections on self-help first-aid for pain, and on home application of the methods discussed.

PART ONE

Pain – what is it?

CHAPTER ONE

Our perception of pain

Only you can measure your own pain. There is no medical or scientific way of objectively telling where your pain is or of knowing how much you are hurting without you providing information on what you feel and where you feel it.

Pain can be described by words or gestures, by body language and facial contortions which give clues as to the site and possibly the degree of what you are feeling but, despite the richness of language, words can only approximate what anyone else feels, as we can see by looking at the words used to describe pain.

Medically several methods are used to help people to give an idea of the *intensity* of what it is they are feeling.

1. A choice of words such as mild, moderate, severe, incapacitating and excruciating (as well as other words of similar meaning and 'weight') are provided, and the person affected chooses the most appropriate one. This can be useful in assessing what they feel to be the intensity of the pain at any given time, but it is not a very sensitive method, and the numerical scale (see below) is more useful.
2. The person affected is told that they should grade their pain between 0 and 10 with 0 equalling no pain at all and ten equalling the most severe pain they can imagine. They are then asked to indicate what number applies to their pain at that moment. This use of numbers is an effective way of recording the difference in perception of pain before and after

McGill Pain Questionnaire

Patient's Name _____ Date _____ Time _____ am/pm

PRI: S _____ A _____ E _____ M _____ PRI(T) _____ PPI _____
      (1-10)   (11-15)   (16)   (17-20)   (1-20)

1 Flickering __
   Quivering __
   Pulsing __
   Throbbing __
   Beating __
   Pounding __

2 Jumping __
   Flashing __
   Shooting __

3 Pricking __
   Boring __
   Drilling __
   Stabbing __
   Lancinating __

4 Sharp __
   Cutting __
   Lacerating __

5 Pinching __
   Pressing __
   Gnawing __
   Cramping __
   Crushing __

6 Tugging __
   Pulling __
   Wrenching __

7 Hot __
   Burning __
   Scalding __
   Searing __

8 Tingling __
   Itchy __
   Smarting __
   Stinging __

9 Dull __
   Sore __
   Hurting __
   Aching __
   Heavy __

10 Tender __
   Taut __
   Rasping __
   Splitting __

11 Tiring __
   Exhausting __

12 Sickening __
   Suffocating __

13 Fearful __
   Frightful __
   Terrifying __

14 Punishing __
   Gruelling __
   Cruel __
   Vicious __
   Killing __

15 Wretched __
   Blinding __

16 Annoying __
   Troublesome __
   Miserable __
   Intense __
   Unbearable __

17 Spreading __
   Radiating __
   Penetrating __
   Piercing __

18 Tight __
   Numb __
   Drawing __
   Squeezing __
   Tearing __

19 Cool __
   Cold __
   Freezing __

20 Nagging __
   Nauseating __
   Agonizing __
   Dreadful __
   Torturing __

PPI
0 No pain __
1 Mild __
2 Discomforting __
3 Distressing __
4 Horrible __
5 Excruciating __

Brief __	Rhythmic __	Continuous __
Momentary __	Periodic __	Steady __
Transient __	Intermittent __	Constant __

E = External
I = Internal

COMMENTS:

treatment. It reveals a lot about how someone feels and the strength of their pain. The approach is similar to one in which people are asked to record the degree of change in previously reported pain – after treatment perhaps – by saying whether its intensity is now the same, half as strong, a quarter as strong, and so on.

3. An analogue scale ('visual analogue scale' or VAS) can be used in which the patient is given a piece of paper with a line either 10 centimetres or 10 inches long drawn on it. The figure 0 is marked at the left end and 10 at the right end, and the patient is asked to mark the line at the point where they feel their pain intensity would be measured if 0 equals no pain and 10 is extreme pain. The length of line to the mark made is measured and this represents the patient's feelings about the intensity of their own perceived pain at that time.

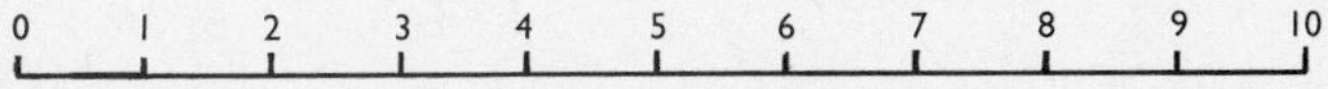

FIGURE 2 A Visual Analogue Scale (VAS).

NOT HOW MUCH BUT WHAT?

Useful as these methods can be, none of them describes the *feeling* or *quality* of the pain. The number and variety of words used to describe pain are quite amazing. Research by Drs Melzack and Torgenson into articles on pain resulted in the choice of over 100 words divided as follows:

FIGURE I The McGill Pain Questionnaire allows the patient to choose the most appropriate description for their pain. Questions 1–10 reflect what the patient feels in relation to the pain; 11–15 reflect the emotional interpretation the patient ascribes to the pain; 16 describes how the patient evaluates the pain in relation to their life at the time; 17–20 provide further descriptions which may be useful. The words chosen are graded as having particular value ('weight') and the total is scored in the space PRI(T). PPI is the patient's evaluation of their 'Present Pain Intensity'. The questionnaire gives a 'snapshot' of the person at the time of interview and is useful for comparison as time goes by and pain improves, or fails to do so.

- *Sensory qualities* such as cramping; aching; pounding; shooting; stabbing; throbbing; tender and sharp
- *Affective qualities* such as tiring; sickening; exhausting; fearful and cruel
- *Evaluative qualities* such as annoying; unbearable and intense
- *Temporal qualities* such as constant or rhythmic.

Research has shown that particular painful conditions result in very similar words being used. For example, it was found that over a third of women suffering from menstrual pain described their pain as cramping; aching; tiring; sickening and constant. Arthritic pain was described as gnawing; aching; exhausting; annoying; constant or rhythmic. Post herpes pain was described variously as sharp; pulling; aching; tender; exhausting; constant or rhythmic. Cancer pain was described as shooting; sharp; gnawing; burning; heavy; exhausting; unbearable; constant or rhythmic.

Clearly there is an overlap in the use of particular words in relation to different conditions, but sometimes very clear evidence of what is going on can be gathered from use of particular words – for example 'gnawing' pain in the fingers indicates probable arthritis, while severe burning pain in the chest could hint at an impending heart attack.

What we learn from this is that the intensity of pain is easily defined, and that language offers a unique way of describing what it is that is being felt. This takes us closer to an awareness of the experience of pain, an as yet unsolved mystery in many ways.

HOW UPBRINGING INFLUENCES YOUR PAIN THRESHOLD

Your pain threshold is the point at which you first begin to feel a sensation from a pain stimulus. This varies from person to person, some people having a much higher pain threshold than others. There are a number of ways of measuring the threshold level – one is by using a heat source (an infra red lamp, for example) placed close to the skin and having the heat slowly increased as the volunteer reports what they feel, saying when they first feel heat and when it becomes painful, and finally when it is too painful to stand. Another way is by the application of an electric shock, at first very mildly and subsequently with escalating intensity as the subject reports reactions. Tests such as this have shown that we all have four different threshold levels, the first of which is the same in almost everyone.

1. The lowest threshold is that of *sensation* alone, and at this point we first experience a feeling – either warmth or a slight tingling from tests such as the ones just mentioned.
2. The second threshold is the one at which *pain is first noticed*.
3. The third is the level at which *pain becomes intolerable*. This is called the higher level, or *tolerance level*, and it is the point at which we say we have had enough and do not want the test to continue.
4. The fourth level is the same as the tolerance level, but one which may be acceptably exceeded if we are successfully encouraged to stand a higher intensity of heat or electrical stimulus.

The level of pain threshold varies between different population and cultural groups. Melzack and Wall report that if electric shock tests are applied to Nepalese subjects they will usually report pain at a far higher level than Europeans tested in the same way, and allow a far greater intensity to be reached before the highest level of tolerance is reached.

When volunteers are encouraged to try to stand a bit more of the 'experimental pain', it has been found to be usually unsuccessful when Mediterranean people of Italian origin are involved, whilst it is frequently successful in Mediterranean people of Jewish origin, and in native Americans. The way the pain is handled emotionally is also different amongst these three example groups, with the Italians demanding instant pain relief, the Jewish people becoming concerned as to the implications of the pain and the native Americans withdrawing into an inner state of calm, indulging in no sound of complaint unless they are quite alone.

In one extraordinary study conducted in 1960, it was shown that Jewish and Protestant groups responded differently after such tests when they were told that the other religious group had shown greater pain tolerance than their group. When they were then retested the Jewish group showed a greatly increased tolerance level, whereas the Protestant group showed no change. There *is*, it seems from this, an inbuilt ability to alter tolerance levels, which is profoundly important in pain treatment.

WHY ARE THERE VARIATIONS?

Attitudes developed in childhood carry forward into adult life. Families which fuss a lot when a child is hurt or cries create a pattern for life in their offspring, just as a different pattern for life emerges from families and cultures in which little notice is taken of minor mishaps.

From experience with battle wounded soldiers it has been found that one in three complain of so much pain that morphine is needed to ease it, whilst others with similar injuries report no pain at all or at least do not need medication to control what they do report. One interpretation of this is that some feel such relief at having been removed from the field of battle that they are not at all shocked by the experience, and the pain from their wounds is thus modified. This is quite likely because it is known that fear, anxiety and worry act to increase the degree of pain perceived, while for those who are relaxed, philosophical and showing no anxiety the opposite tends to be the case.

Pain that occurs during intense sporting activity is often not felt as pain because the person is so focused on other things that they may not be aware of even severe injury until later on. Similarly people with chronic pain often learn to focus attention on to an activity which diverts them from the pain's intensity. This technique is useful only when pain is constant or rising in intensity slowly, not when it changes rapidly.

A sense of control over pain also changes how intensely it is felt, and a number of techniques, including learning relaxation methods and self-application of instruments which ease the pain can help to achieve this sense of control.

Pain threshold can be influenced by other factors as well, including the amazing power of suggestion (as in hypnosis and self-hypnosis) and the little understood power of the placebo.

So, it can be seen that what you believe pain to mean, how much attention you are giving to it, or to other matters, as well as the sort of society/culture/family in which you were brought up, will all influence the way you handle pain. The fact that the way you see pain can often be changed by the use of special techniques is particularly important should you ever be faced with chronic pain.

CHAPTER TWO

Getting to grips with pain

Pain is, therefore, both a physical and psychological experience, and the degree of pain you feel is influenced by many factors, not least your social and cultural background. The way you sense pain is also influenced by the degree of anxiety associated with it, and one of the key elements in the psychological approach to pain relief is to understand the nature of it. Why is the pain there? What is actually happening? Suffering pain without knowing the cause adds to anxiety, and once a diagnosis has been made – even if it means accepting bad news – at least the nature of the enemy is known and strategies can be devised to reduce its power.

Knowledge alone is not enough, though, and coping or control skills need to be learned to overcome the feeling of powerlessness that can develop. Understanding the pain is important so that the emotional undertones that are associated with it can be fully appreciated, and to reach a level of control and understanding often calls for skilled counselling and, perhaps, psychotherapy.

It is a fact that when attention is turned to a pain being suffered it is felt more acutely, and that a preoccupying distraction can 'take your mind off it' to the extent that you feel it much less, or are unaware of feeling it. Many people with chronic pain conditions help themselves by focusing on activities such as listening to music or some intricate hobby which takes them away from the pain. The acceptance of known 'positive' pain, such as may occur in childbirth, can be further assisted by distraction, and this is where breathing exercises and conscious relaxation efforts can help.

Distraction, however, is only really successful when pain is static or increasing very slowly. It does not seem to work when pain changes rapidly.

THE CONTROL FACTOR

The three elements in pain reduction – understanding the pain, anxiety reduction and distraction – are all greatly helped by having a sense of control over the pain. With such a sense of control (anything which modifies the pain) comes a feeling of no longer being at the mercy of the pain process, but of having some influence and power over it. You can learn to exercise control by using one or more of the self-help techniques described in this book, and once you acquire a sense of control over the pain there is usually a rapid drop in anxiety levels, and the pain will be felt less intensely.

PSYCHOTHERAPY

Where chronic pain exists there is much to be said for skilled psychotherapy which helps the person affected to deal more effectively with their problem, and numerous techniques have evolved for use in such cases.

These include what are called cognitive strategies, or attempts to unravel the emotional aspects of a person's pain. This may involve two key areas of the problem – the subjective way they are experiencing and 'suffering' the pain, and their response to the pain . . . what they are doing about it. It is often also necessary to sort out just what the pain means in your life. Does it carry with it an inability to work, thus adding to stress? Or does it provide an escape from relationships or tasks which you are glad to be free of, thus reducing your stress load?

Skilled counselling may be needed in some cases of chronic pain, but the formula of anxiety reduction/distraction/control offers most sufferers from pain a way forward as they learn to adapt to what may be a permanent situation.

UNDERSTANDING THE 'GATE' THEORY OF PAIN

For thousands of years before Melzack and Wall produced their research findings explaining how pain is transmitted in the body (known as the 'gate' theory) the Chinese unknowingly exploited it whenever they used acupuncture in treating pain.

At its simplest this theory describes how one sensation (such as touch or vibration) can mask another, and how, when that other sensation is pain, this can be a valuable way of relieving it. From the beginning of time people have instinctively known the benefits of rubbing a painful area. The rubbing applies a light and rapid pressure, a sort of high frequency/low intensity movement, which masks the pain. When an acupuncture needle is used to treat pain it is inserted and rotated slowly, and this can be described as a low frequency/high intensity movement. Both are effective, so if we look at how sensations caused by these actions are transmitted we should be able to discover how they block pain.

The nerve fibres which are activated by rubbing are the same as those which become active through vibration and electrical stimulation using TENS machines (small units which pass a mild current across painful regions to mask the pain). Rubbing, and some aspects of acupuncture, depend on extremely rapid transmission along special low-threshold (easily stimulated) *fast* nerve fibres while pain is carried slowly along fibres with a higher threshold (more difficult to stimulate). This means that if the fast (sensation) fibres can be stimulated the messages they carry will effectively 'shut the gate' to the pain messages before (and possibly after) they enter the spinal cord for transmission up to the brain.

The pain messages can also be influenced by other features of the way acupuncture is used (rotation and electrical stimulation of needles, for example) which causes the release of natural pain-killing substances called endorphins. Research has also shown that direct finger pressure on acupuncture points releases endorphins, which explains many of the benefits of acupressure and other oriental massage methods.

There are also influences downwards from the brain which can reduce pain perception and greatly alter the amount of pain felt. For example, a pain which is thought to be 'productive', such as one that may be experienced in childbirth, is likely to be much more readily acceptable than one which has no positive aspects.

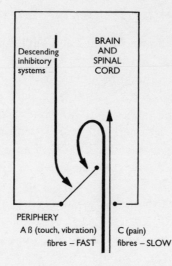

FIGURE 3 Pain fibres open the gate into the central nervous system, but this gate can be partly or completely shut, either from the inside, through the influence of the mind (as, say, in the case of a soldier wounded during battle), or from the outside, by inhibitory mechanisms such as the sensation of acupuncture, touch or vibration.

This simplified outline of the 'gate' theory does not do full justice to the highly complex mechanisms at work, but it gives an idea of the way that we can exploit the natural features of the nervous system (different speeds of transmission of different sensations, with pain being on the slow train; as well as the natural pain-killers which our bodies have handy in case of pain). It also helps to put into perspective the overall influence of the mind by which we can manipulate the 'gate' mechanism according to what we think and believe about the pain we are experiencing.

New discoveries are emerging from research which show that nerves carry not just messages which we can think of as electrical transmissions but also (fairly slowly) substances including proteins and fatty acids. These have major effects on the tissues which the nerve supplies and also the way various 'junction boxes' (synapses) along its route behave, influencing the passage of electrical messages, making them either faster or slower.

The ways in which acupuncture and other milder stimulants, such as massage, electrical stimulation etc., can influence the movement of these substances along the nerves is still being researched and is bound to enlarge our understanding of how pain can be modified.

PART TWO

Pain relief – how you can achieve it

CHAPTER THREE

Current orthodox approaches to pain

Implicit in good medicine is the need to find the cause of pain before attempting pain-killing methods, but this can sometimes go unheeded, especially in self-treatment, so that pain is dealt with as though it is the totality of the problem rather than the symptom. Pain can have outlived its usefulness, or be the result of uncomplicated causes, but it can also be a warning of a developing serious problem. Finding out which of these is the case is the job of a trained physician. Self-diagnosis is therefore not recommended.

There are, of course, cases when heroic measures are called for – when pain is so severe that it demands immediate attention. Also, the desperate desire to do something quickly when someone helpless is in pain – such as a young child who cannot tell you where it hurts – can lead to pain relief being given priority over finding the cause. In such situations it is very important that whatever is done should not make things worse by producing side-effects. Some of the commonest orthodox approaches to pain relief seem to carry risks, especially when used by non-professionals, and it is even possible that under pressure to do something – anything – to help someone in pain, a doctor might resort to symptomatic treatment rather than get involved in a time-consuming and often frustrating search for causes.

ATTACKING PAIN WITH DRUGS

As a general rule, orthodox medicine deals with pain in a progressively aggressive manner, using drugs as its main weapon. Mild drugs, many of which are available over the counter without prescription (such as aspirin) are almost universally used against pain as a first line of attack.

Aspirin and similar drugs are effective because they interfere with a process at the site of some painful conditions, and block the series of events which lead to pain. This apparently desirable effect is, however, very often accompanied by serious undesirable ones. If such mild analgesic (pain deadening) drugs should fail, stronger ones such as codeine might be tried or, if the condition involves inflammation, an anti-inflammatory drug might be used, including those which are based on cortisone (a hormonal or steroid drug).

THE NSAID SAGA

For many years, until quite recently, a major treatment of the pain of osteoarthritis was a series of anti-inflammatory drugs. Those which were not cortisone-based were known as 'non-steroidal anti-inflammatory drugs', or NSAIDs. They were effective in reducing inflammation and pain in many cases, but the true cost in terms of side-effects has only recently become apparent. It had long been recognized that there was a risk of bleeding in the stomach, but not the possibility that the arthritic condition of those receiving the drugs was actually likely to become worse than if no treatment had been given, with damaged joints deteriorating dramatically.

This is largely because the inflammatory processes are themselves part of the body's defence and repair mechanism, and it has now been shown that when these processes are interfered with by NSAIDs – although patients feel better for a while – in the long run even worse arthritis might develop. When cortisone type medication is used this is also true, but the side-effects tend to be worse.

WHEN IN DOUBT TRANQUILLIZE!

In cases of intractable pain it is common for anti-depressant medication (tranquillizers) to be used, since when anxiety is reduced pain is not felt as strongly. Unfortunately these drugs can become addictive, and their use for anything but a short time is now thought to be undesirable by much of orthodox medicine. If the cause of pain lies in the musculoskeletal system, muscle relaxant medication might also be used, although research evidence suggests that this approach is not always very effective.

NARCOTIC DRUGS

If there is still strong pain despite the use of any or all of the first and second line methods, the really serious drugs – opiates such as morphine – might be used. These are effective because they mimic the action of the natural pain-killers which the body itself produces. They attach to the receptor sites in the central nervous system and brain which are prepared to receive our own endorphins.

The much publicized problems of addiction and subsequent withdrawal symptoms, associated in most people's minds with medical use of opiates, is thought by leading researchers such as Drs Melzack and Wall to be grossly over-exaggerated, especially when they are used for a short time only. Sometimes such problems are mild, they state, but more often they are not even noticed.

All of the above approaches carry some risk of unpleasant and sometimes serious reactions.

OTHER PAIN-KILLING METHODS

In some instances relief from pain is attempted by the surgical destruction of nerve pathways, or of parts of the central nervous system – even parts of the brain in certain cases. Most of this is dangerous, and there is a high failure rate. Not only is surgery such as this likely to fail to relieve the pain being treated, but it commonly creates new pain, and these methods are largely an act of desperation. As Drs Melzack and Wall state in their book

The Challenge of Pain: 'Long-term control of pain is rarely achieved by surgery.' While they support its use in cases where the patient is in much pain and has only a short time to live, its use in other situations is, they believe, 'often a disaster'.

The use of deep x-ray treatment to deal with the chronic pain associated with some forms of cancer is similar to surgical procedures in that it is of possible benefit in the short-term, but with little to say for it in the long term.

MIND ORIENTED METHODS

To its credit, orthodox medicine is well aware of many of the shortcomings of the methods outlined here, and it has developed a range of coping and counselling strategies which are extremely effective in helping people with chronic pain. Unfortunately these are seldom used outside specialist pain clinics because they are time consuming and largely inappropriate for general practice settings.

In orthodox pain clinics some of the best of the skilful use of drug control is combined with the use of psychological and relaxation/anti-anxiety methods, together with an increasing use of some of the alternative strategies such as acupuncture and physical medicine. Later in the book I describe some of these methods, many of which are suitable for self-application, especially a number of easily learned relaxation and breathing techniques.

ALTERNATIVES

Finding the balance between good effects and side-effects of treatment is the real art of healing. All too often, with the best intentions, short-term drug and surgical measures aimed at relieving pain make matters worse because this balance is not found. Fortunately, there are other less dangerous ways of using the body's natural pain-killing mechanisms which the opiate drugs exploit, without having to resort to drugs (acupuncture and acupressure are good alternatives).

There are also more 'natural' ways of interfering with the inflammatory processes which accompany some forms of pain, using simple and safe nutritional means (although this is not always a good idea because inflammation is part of the body's defence reaction); and there are, of course, many better ways of achieving relaxation than by using tranquillizers.

Natural pain relief, without the use of drugs, may therefore be a real possibility in many cases.

CHAPTER FOUR

Nutritional control of inflammation

Pain can be reduced or controlled in a number of ways:

1. By reducing or masking the sending of the pain messages.
2. By reducing the intensity of those messages.
3. By, in some way, blocking the messages.
4. By changing the way the messages are interpreted once they have been received by the central nervous system and brain.

Where inflammation is a part of the cause of the pain it is possible to bring about a reduction in pain transmission (item 1. above) by using safe methods which reduce the inflammation. Remember that many pain-killing drugs, such as aspirin, do just this, but unfortunately almost all of them have side-effects, some of which can be serious.

There are two major nutritional anti-inflammatory methods which can prove effective in most cases of pain suffering. One is the dietary approach, and the other is the enzyme approach. Both or either can be used where appropriate.

WHEN ARE THESE METHODS APPROPRIATE?

Inflammation is a natural and mostly useful response by the body to irritation, injury and infection. It can be a major part of the process of getting better despite the fact that it is not particularly pleasant. So, to drastically alter or reduce inflammation may be counterproductive, and you should discuss things with a health care professional to ascertain that this is a safe way forward before putting nutritional inflammation reducing tactics into action.

If pain is reduced by these methods, or by any others, it is a mistake to take it as a licence to become very active if this is stressing a previously inflamed or damaged joint or area. Remember that overuse of damaged joint surfaces is one of the reasons why arthritis can get worse over time when the pain is continually eased by drugs. It is always safer to seek professional advice rather than to try things for yourself and simply hope for the best.

DIETARY TACTICS

Reduce intake of animal fats

A major part of pain and inflammation processes involves minute chemical substances, which your body makes, called prostaglandins and leukotrienes. These are themselves to a great extent dependent upon the presence of arachidonic acid which the human system manufactures mainly from animal fats. So, by reducing animal fat intake, this cuts down your access to the enzymes which help to produce arachidonic acid, and this in turn cuts down the levels of the inflammatory substances which, when released in tissues, contribute so greatly to pain.

This, then, is the first priority in an anti-inflammatory dietary approach – cut down or eliminate dietary fat. Fat-free or low-fat milk, yogurt and cheese should be used in preference to full-fat varieties, and butter should be avoided altogether. Meat fat should be completely avoided, and since much fat in meat is invisible, meat itself could be left out of the diet for a time (or permanently). Poultry skin should not be eaten. Information on packaging should be scrutinized for hidden fats in manufactured food items such as biscuits.

Eat fish and increase fish oil intake

Some fish, mainly that which comes from cold water areas such as the North Sea, contain high levels of eicosapentenoic acid (EPA) which reduces levels of arachidonic acid in tissues and therefore helps to modify the release of inflammatory substances in the body. The most important thing about fish oil is that whilst it has an anti-inflammatory effect it does not interfere with the beneficial activity of the prostaglandins, such as the protection of delicate stomach lining and the maintenance of the correct blood clotting levels.

There are many drugs which can do what fish oil can do (reduce inflammation and thereafter pain) but only at the risk of causing new problems – something EPA does not do, unless you are allergic to fish. Research has shown that the use of EPA in rheumatic and arthritic conditions can offer relief from swelling, stiffness and pain; although benefits do not usually become evident until after at least three months of supplementation, with the best effects showing after six months.

To use this strategy you should eat fish such as herring, sardine, salmon and mackerel at least twice weekly, and more frequently if you wish. At the same time take 10–15 (standard size) EPA capsules daily.

Amino acids: phenylalanine (DLPA)

Amino acids are protein fractions which are a natural part of our bodies, and which our bodies use to manufacture new tissues and cells. When taken individually they can have special effects, as is the case with DLPA (DL-Phenylalanine) which has been shown to have pain-killing potential under certain circumstances – for example, when a person is having some other form of treatment such as pain-killing drugs or having acupuncture. On its own it does not seem to have much effect, but it acts in the form of a catalyst when used as an adjunct to other treatments. Doses recommended are from 2 to 3 grams daily in divided doses taken between meals.

Anti-inflammatory enzymes

Enzymes are minute chemical substances which take part in biochemical reactions in our bodies. Some, such as protease, are closely involved in the digestion of protein (proteolytic enzymes), and it has been found that the use of protein-digesting enzymes derived from plants has a gentle but substantial anti-inflammatory effect. These plant enzymes include bromelaine (from the pineapple plant) and papain (from the papaya plant). Health Food stores and pharmacies sell them. It is necessary to take between 2 and 3 grams of one or the other (bromelaine is more effective), spread throughout the day, but between meals, as part of an anti-inflammatory pain relieving strategy.

Don't drink instant coffee

It has been found that coffee contains substances which block the receptor sites used by our natural pain-killing endorphins, making pain seem more intense. This seems only to be the case with instant coffee as against brewed forms of coffee. This is not a recommendation to drink brewed coffee, but a suggestion that at least instant coffee should be avoided by those in pain.

SPECIFIC NUTRIENTS FOR SPECIFIC PAINS

In some instances special needs demand particular nutrients to help. For example, in cases of painful muscle cramping, the use of magnesium and calcium may be helpful, and the problems of premenstrual syndrome have been found to be alleviated by the use of evening primrose oil, vitamins E and B6 and magnesium.

CHAPTER FIVE

Counter-irritation methods, acupuncture and TENS

Centuries of use of different pain-control methods became 'respectable' when Melzack and Wall explained their 'gate' theory in 1965. This explained scientifically how low level stimulation could slow down or stop transmission of pain messages, and how more intense stimulation could 'shut the gate', and that these things happened because of mechanisms involving the nervous system and brain.

Acupuncture and acupressure thus became acceptable to doctors, and some of the ways massage works became clearer. Also, new methods of treatment, such as TENS, were developed.

TENS EXPLAINED

When TENS is used, two small pads are attached to the skin overlying or on each side of a painful area, with a gel (to improve electrical contact) between the pads and the skin. A mild electrical current from a tiny battery-operated unit is passed between the pads with its intensity usually under the direct control of the person with the pain. This allows the patient to turn up the current until they feel a pleasant tingling sensation which effectively masks their pain by stimulating all nerves up to an inch and a half (approx 4 cms) below the skin on which the pads lie.

TENS has been shown in trial after trial to be most effective in chronic pain control, although it works in acute pain as well. Best results are

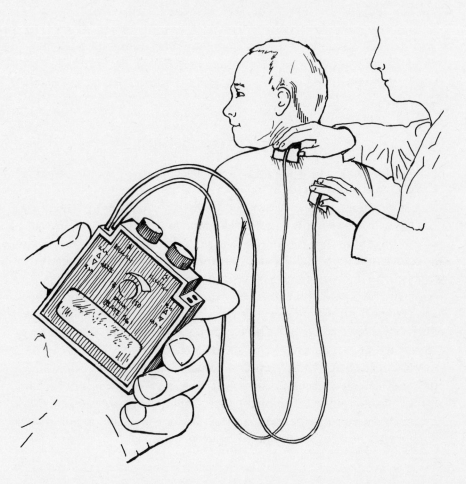

FIGURE 4 TENS machines produce a mild electrical current controlled by the patient which can be effective in the control of both chronic and acute pain.

achieved when there are painful muscle areas involved, or where the skin over the painful area is sensitive, especially when this is associated with local nerve damage.

The results of TENS have been found to be far superior to those achieved by dummy (placebo) machines. There are absolutely no side-effects, and it has become the first treatment choice of almost all pain clinics worldwide because it is safe, effective and relatively inexpensive. Units cost between

£40 and £150 depending upon how sophisticated they are.

Of great importance to people with chronic pain conditions is the fact that in many cases the relief felt lasts long after the machine has been switched off, and also that there is frequently a rise in the threshold at which pain is felt.

VARIABLE FACTORS

Where the contact pads are placed can make all the difference between success and failure of pain relief with TENS machines, and some experimentation may be necessary to find which positions give the most relief. The usual advice is to place them one on either side, or above and below, the painful area. Ideally you should try to find areas where the skin or muscle feels more tender than surrounding areas and try these first. There are two other very important variables in TENS application, apart from where the pads should be sited – one is the intensity of the impulses, and the other is the frequency of these. If you think of frequency as how often waves of electrical impulses are sent and of intensity as how strong these waves are, you can see that quite different sensations can be achieved by varying them. Anything from slow deep impulses to rapid shallow ones, or any other combination imaginable, is possible. What seems important is that whatever intensity and frequency is used, the sensation should be tolerable or even pleasant, and that it should mask the pain or completely abolish it, at least while the unit is switched on.

DIFFERENT PROBLEMS – DIFFERENT SETTINGS

In rheumatoid arthritis, pain is relieved more effectively and for longer when high frequency (70Hz) is used compared with low frequency (3Hz). When patients with pain from nervous system damage are treated some are helped by high frequency and some by low frequency applications of TENS. Trial and error in this as well as placement of the pads is called for to get the best results.

ADVANTAGES OF TENS

1. Safety is absolute unless a pain is being masked which should receive attention.
2. When pain is reduced (and sometimes it goes altogether during the period that TENS is used) tense muscles may relax allowing more normal use during and after its application.
3. TENS provides users with a degree of *control* over their condition, perhaps for the first time. This is of immense importance in chronic pain conditions.

Probably the only negative comment to be made about TENS is that referred to in 1. above, namely that its use might prevent someone from dealing with the cause of their problem – but this is true of all methods of pain relief.

ACUPUNCTURE AND ACUPRESSURE

Acupuncture involves the use of needles or heat (known as moxibustion) to stimulate or sedate special points on the body surface for various effects, including pain relief, and it is very effective in this. We now know that a combination of control of the 'gate' mechanism and the release of natural pain-killing substances (endorphins/enkephalins) produces the remarkable benefits which this system delivers. There is undoubtedly a placebo effect as well, but this is so with most treatment methods, and should not in any way detract from the respect that acupuncture deserves.

It has been found that all the known trigger points are mapped in acupuncture as points for use in treatment. Pressure on these (as used in acupressure or Shiatsu) has been shown to produce as much and sometimes more pain relief compared with the use of needles.

OTHER WAYS OF STIMULATING POINTS

Similar pain relief has also been achieved using lasers, electrical stimulation and injections on or into acupuncture points. What this tells us is that there are many ways of reflexively influencing these sensitive points, all of which can bring in to play the combined influences of the blocking or reduction of pain messages and the release of pain-killing hormones by the body. Clearly, acupuncture itself is not a do-it-yourself therapy, but acupressure certainly can be, and the methods used are the same as those suggested for self-treating trigger points.

There are available, though, small electric stimulation machines which can be used to find and treat active acupuncture points. They find these by measuring electrical resistance of the skin which is lower when a point is 'active' (at which time it will also be more sensitive to pressure). By pressing a button a small electric impulse is then delivered to the point.

PATTERNS OF POINTS FOR TREATMENT

Interestingly, it is not always necessary to use points close to the site of pain in acupuncture, electro-acupuncture or acupressure. In many cases distant points are useful, as are points on the surface of the ear and on the opposite side of the body (left knee treated for pain in the right, for example).

The general rules for use of acupuncture points for pain relief are as follows:

- points are treated which encircle the painful area, or
- a line of points along a limb may be treated, and/or
- points distant to the pain as well as local to it are treated, and/or
- points on the same side as the pain as well as those on the opposite side of the body are employed, and/or
- points on the auricle (outer ear) are used.

HOW TO FIND THE POINTS TO PRESS IN ACUPRESSURE

Acupuncture points which are reflexively active are tender to pressure. This means that anything that hurts when you press it is for that moment suitable for acupuncture/acupressure. Sometimes, however, the repetitive pressing needed to find the tenderness is more than you might wish to put up with, if you are already in enough pain.

Other ways of finding the suitable points include:

- Use of electrical detection devices as mentioned above.
- Lightly running a finger (feather-light touch) over the skin. Wherever there is a sense of 'drag' or where the passage of the finger is in some way less easy, there is probable reflex activity under the skin, and this might prove sensitive on light pressure.
- By lightly stretching the skin apart, using index fingers to assess its elasticity, and comparing this with the skin alongside in a series of rapid stretches, wherever the elastic quality is reduced there is likely to be reflex activity underneath that patch of skin.

WHAT TO DO TO THE POINTS

Once found, acupressure can be applied to the points by a steady, deep but not hurtful pressure for 10 to 20 seconds at a time. A series of points treated in this way or by electro-acupuncture around or along, or on opposite sides, of painful sites will frequently produce marked pain relief, albeit temporarily.

No-one should ever try self-application of acupuncture using needles. This is a specialized method and a professional should be consulted.

OTHER METHODS OF COUNTER-IRRITATION

The use of ice or heat in treating pain also brings into play some of the nerve responses which are used in acupuncture and acupressure, as do the 'hot' substances found in herbal rubs derived from paprika or chili peppers (see the section on herbal methods of treating pain).

Other methods which are used in some societies include cupping (use of heated cups which are placed over spinal and other areas to produce a vacuum suction), as well as scarification (minute cuts of the skin with a fine blade), cauterization (burning hot applications to specific areas) and blistering techniques using irritant substances.

All of these have their advocates, and seem to use a sort of hyper-stimulation which overloads or blocks pain transmission, but none of them should be attempted as self-treatment.

CHAPTER SIX

Pain relief through stress reduction

There is a great deal of evidence which shows that it is possible to reduce the amount of pain you are feeling by altering the degree of what is called 'arousal'. In simple terms, if you have a chronically painful condition, the more anxious you are the more easily aroused you will be, and the more pain you will feel. The less anxious you are, the less easily aroused you will be and the less pain you will feel, at least in relation to chronic pain.

HOW DO DOCTORS MEASURE AROUSAL?

There are a number of ways of assessing your arousal, including measurement of the electrical resistance of your skin, or the amount of activity in key muscles when you are resting, or the type of brain-wave activity most common in your brain.

You can easily recognize that your arousal levels are high when you develop any of the following signs:

- Being more restless and/or easily upset than usual
- Having difficulty in relaxing
- Disturbed sleep pattern
- Sighing a lot, or breathing more shallowly than usual
- Having difficulty in concentrating
- Feeling on edge
- An almost constant sense of anxiety

WHAT'S TO BE DONE?

If being aroused indicates that you are anxious and that whatever pain you are aware of is being felt more strongly than is necessary, what can you do about it?

Part of the answer is to learn to reduce your anxiety level, and this is surprisingly easy in many cases. You can start from a number of different places in order to achieve this. All will lead to the same result if successful – a reduction in arousal/anxiety and a lessening of the level of pain you are feeling.

1. *Breathing*: You can start by learning a simple traditional Yoga breathing method which has been shown in medical studies to lower arousal/anxiety states very quickly. Everyone in pain should learn to do this. Instructions are given in this chapter.

2. *Biofeedback*: You can use a small machine which measures your skin resistance, your temperature (of a hand possibly) or your muscle tension (or perhaps your blood pressure) and which, by means of sound, screen or dial, shows the level of whatever is being measured. The idea is to try to change/learn to control at will the level shown – make a high pitched sound lower, the waveform on a screen flatter, or the needle on a dial move – by conscious effort. Any success in this is immediately registered by the machine, and therefore enables the user to effectively focus further effort. In this way people have learned to lower their blood pressure, to improve circulation to legs or arms, to 'switch off' migraine headaches, to slow or speed up their heart rate and to control pain – at will. Along with TENS, biofeedback has become one of the most used methods in pain clinics and hospitals which deal with pain.

3. *Relaxation*: You can use one of a great many methods of relaxation. These have much the same effect as biofeedback, but without using a machine. Relaxation techniques can take longer to reduce arousal than biofeedback, but they are likely to be just as successful in the long run, and are usually more successful for that small but significant percentage of people who do not do well with biofeedback because of a resistance to working with machines.

4. *Visualization*: You can use what is called visualization or guided imagery. This produces very similar results to both relaxation and biofeedback.

THE QUESTION OF SLEEP

Sufferers from chronic pain frequently experience sleep disturbance, and this serves to compound the pain problem by increasing anxiety and stress levels. The vicious circle which develops starts with pain which produces fear and anxiety and a sense of powerlessness and helplessness, and this leads to sleep difficulties which in turn feed into the whole cycle, compounding it and making everything seem worse; increasing arousal and escalating the pain.

ANTI-AROUSAL BREATHING TECHNIQUE

There are many exercises to help improve breathing, but there is just one which has been shown in medical studies to effectively reduce arousal and anxiety levels. This is an exercise based on traditional yogic pranayama breathing.

The pattern is as follows:

1. Having placed yourself in a comfortable (ideally seated) position, you inhale fully while counting to yourself up to no more than three (ideally two). Translated into practical terms, this means that you fill your lungs fairly quickly. The counting is necessary because the timing of the inhalation and exhalation phase of breathing is critical in this exercise.
2. Without pausing to hold your breath, you then exhale fully, taking four, five or even six seconds to do so (count to yourself at the same speed as when you inhaled).
3. Repeat the inhalation (two seconds) and the exhalation. The object is that, in time and with practice, you should make this exhalation phase last eight seconds.
4. All inhalation should be through the nose if possible, while exhalation can be through nose or mouth. Most important is that your breathing out must be slow and continuous. It is no use breathing the air out in two seconds and then simply waiting until the count reaches five or six before inhaling again.
5. Repeat the cycles of inhalation/exhalation for several minutes with a least six cycles per minute (each cycle should eventually last ten

seconds – two in and eight out – although at first you may find two in/three or four out is all you can manage). By the time you have completed ten or so cycles your sense of anxiety should be much reduced, and your awareness of pain lessened.

6. Do this exercise every hour *if you are anxious, or whenever pain or anxiety/stress seem to be building up.*

FOCUS ON BREATHING MUSCLES

Before doing the exercise described above sit or stand in front of a mirror and observe your shoulders as you breathe deeply. Do they rise towards your ears as you inhale? If so, you are using certain muscles which attach to your neck and shoulders, as well as the upper ribs, in a way which should only happen when you are or have been exerting yourself. To use them when seated or standing shows they are overworking and this will influence your breathing mechanics in a negative way.

To retrain yourself out of this habit (that is all it is) and help reduce the related tendency to hyperventilate (which increases anxiety/arousal levels) you should do the following exercise, either separately from the routine above or as part of it.

1. Sit in a chair which has arms, and rest your arms on the chair.
2. As you practise deep breathing, make sure your elbows are firmly pressed downwards towards the floor, against the arms of the chair.

That is all there is to the exercise since while pressing down with your elbows it is impossible to use the muscles which you were previously using, and you are obliged to use correct breathing muscles. Do this at the same time as the rhythmic breathing described above, or at another time until you can sit in front of a mirror and inhale without your shoulders lifting towards your ears.

BIOFEEDBACK

If you can learn a technique which helps you to gain control of specific functions of your body over which you normally have little or no conscious control (your blood pressure, for example) you have every chance of being able to use this skill in easing and managing pain – this is what biofeedback offers.

Biofeedback is best learnt from an expert such as a physiotherapist who specializes in pain or rehabilitation medicine, or a doctor who is experienced in its use, or a psychologist. It is not easy to teach yourself the basic skills, although ultimately you are entirely alone with your machine in learning the techniques which control particular functions.

To be successful you need determination, patience and the right sort of machine to give you the information you need. Failure is usually because of lack of persistence or because of difficulty in relaxing. It is often useful to learn breathing and relaxation methods before starting biofeedback.

BIOFEEDBACK'S GREATEST SUCCESS

The most successful and researched area of pain control using biofeedback relates to headache, both the tension type (a 60 per cent success rate when relaxation and biofeedback methods are used) and migraine (35 per cent success with biofeedback alone, rising to 65 per cent when combined with Autogenic Training – see below). A particular bonus is that the improvements tend to continue long after (for at least a year) ceasing the active use of a biofeedback machine.

Success rates similar to those in dealing with headaches have been shown in Raynaud's disease, torticollis (neck muscle spasm), childbirth, menstrual pain, writer's cramp, duodenal ulcer, kidney infection pain, rheumatoid arthritis, phantom limb pain, angina, TMJ (jaw) problems and pain following trauma.

BIOFEEDBACK MACHINES

A variety of units exist which measure and display different sorts of information for biofeedback purposes.

- Those which measure the degree of tension in the muscles are thought to be the best for use by anyone with musculoskeletal aches and pains

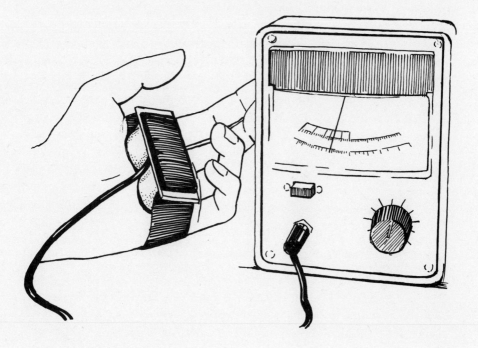

FIGURE 5 A biofeedback machine.

or tension-type headaches, since it leads to direct relaxation of the muscles.

- People with pain associated with circulatory imbalances (intermittent claudication, Raynaud's disease, and migraine, for example) are most likely to benefit from monitors which measure blood flow in some way.
- Biofeedback training involving both muscle tension and circulation makes for a very powerful degree of control over functions which influence most forms of pain. Many people learn one and then the other (sometimes using a unit which can measure and monitor both).
- Biofeedback which monitors brain-waves is most helpful for overall stress, anxiety and arousal reduction, which will help deal with chronic pain in a general way.
- Units which monitor skin resistance to electricity are probably the cheapest available. Learning to alter this feature (electrical resistance) helps achieve lowering of arousal levels as well.

Whichever form you use there will be a marked degree of general benefit, and it has been shown that when you learn to control one feature (say muscle tone) all the others (circulation, brain-wave pattern and electrical resistance) will improve to an extent. Many people find that they can learn quite easily to modify one of these elements but not the others, so if when learning biofeedback techniques you find you are not progressing very fast using one form (say trying to control muscle tension) try another (say circulation).

Most people can eventually learn to alter at least one of their internal processes with great benefit in terms of pain and stress reduction.

RELAXATION TECHNIQUE
(MODIFIED AUTOGENIC TRAINING)

There is general agreement amongst experts that biofeedback and relaxation techniques are equally effective for treating almost all forms of pain. There are a vast number of relaxation exercises, but one in particular (Autogenic Training) comes close to duplicating the benefits of biofeedback, without using machines. It is also quite suitable for self-treatment. Other forms of relaxation are also encouraged, since anything which produces a reduction of muscular tension and mental anxiety can only help relieve chronic pain.

Although Autogenic Training is best learned from a fully trained instructor, the following modified form is an excellent way of achieving some degree of control over muscle tone and/or circulation, and therefore over pain.

1. Lie on the floor or bed in a comfortable position with a small cushion under your head (knees bent if that makes your back feel easier) and your eyes closed.
2. Focus attention on your right hand/arm and silently say to yourself 'my right hand (or arm) feels heavy'. Try to see your arm relaxed and heavy, its weight sinking into the surface it is resting on. Feel its weight. Over a period of about a minute repeat the affirmation several times and try to stay focused on the weight and heaviness of your hand/arm. You will almost certainly lose focus as your attention wanders from time to time.

This is part of the training in the exercise – to stay focused – so don't feel angry, just go back to the hand or arm and its heaviness.

You may or may not be able to sense the heaviness – it doesn't matter too much at first. If you do, stay with it and enjoy the sense of release – of letting go – that comes with it.

3. Next, focus on your left hand/arm and do exactly the same thing for about a minute.

4. Move to your left leg, and then your right leg, with similar timing, messages and focused attention.

5. Go back to your right hand/arm and affirm a message which tells you that you sense a greater degree of warmth there: 'my hand is feeling warm (or hot).'

6. After a minute or so, go to your left hand/arm, your left leg and then finally your right leg, each time with the warming message and attention. If warmth is sensed, stay with it for a while and feel it spread – and enjoy it.

7. Finally, focus on your forehead and affirm that it feels cool and refreshed. Stay with this for a minute before completing the exercise.

By repeating the whole exercise at least once a day (10 to 15 minutes is all it will take) you will gradually find you can stay focused on each region and sensation (heaviness, warmth, coolness) for the full minute in each case.

When you have achieved this (perhaps after a month of daily repetition of the exercises) you will have come close to achieving exactly the degree of control over muscle tension and circulation as you would have done using a biofeedback machine.

'Heaviness' represents what you feel when muscles relax, 'warmth' is what you feel when your circulation to an area is increased, while 'coolness' is the opposite, a reduced circulation for a short while.

VISUALIZATION

What this offers you in pain control terms is of enormous value:

1. If you have pain related to muscle tension you can use the training to

focus on the area, and by getting that area to 'feel' heavy you will reduce tension.

2. If you have pain related to poor circulation you can use the 'warmth' instruction to improve it in any area you wish (a skin thermometer shows an increase of up to a degree when an area is 'made' warmer in Autogenic Training).

3. If you have an inflammation related to your pain you can reduce this by thinking the area 'cool'.

4. You can use the new skills you have learned to focus on any area you wish – and most important, stay focused – and introduce other images, 'seeing' in your mind's eye an ulcer healing, or a stiff joint easing and moving, or a congested swollen area just melting back to normality – or any other helpful change which would ease whatever pain problem you might have.

When you are doing this you are, in fact, practising visualization, or guided imagery. Visualization is usually part of a programme which follows on from deep relaxation, and which asks you to use mental pictures in which harmonious, uplifting and safe images (a sunlit meadow by a sparkling stream, or a quiet beach scene, or a favourite garden or room, for example) are used to produce a profound state of contentment.

The next stage is to direct your mind to encouraging healing of one sort or another. Once imagination has been cultivated in the search for pain relief you can become extremely creative. People have eased their pain by visualizing it in a wide variety of ways, and the use of comic-strip images can be helpful:

- Sharp knife-like pain may be imagined as icy spikes which visualization melts.
- Oppressive pressure pain can be seen as the weight of something extremely heavy which visualization makes thinner and lighter until it floats away.
- Pain of any sort can be thought of as resulting from a science-fiction creature which can be killed by using rays from the brain.
- Pain in a joint which has seized up can be seen being flooded with fresh clear shiny lubrication and so become free again.
- Pain may be seen in your mind's eye as bright red with the visualization

exercise gradually fading this to pink and then white as the pain vanishes along with the colour.

RELAXATION MUST COME FIRST

Whatever visualization image you construct, it is absolutely essential that relaxation is achieved first – and this brings us back to the methods which will help you to relax, such as Autogenic Training and biofeedback.

Visualization adds just one more dimension to these, allowing your mind to become involved more actively in gaining control over pain, and this element of control is extremely important psychologically.

HYPNOSIS

Hypnosis has been found to be effective in treating acute pain (burns, for example) as well as chronic pain where there is a clear understanding of the source of the pain (arthritis or cancer, for example). Success depends on the degree of hypnotic responsiveness of the person receiving it, as well as on a good rapport with the practitioner using it.

Self-hypnosis can be learned by some people as a method of gaining a sense of control over it. The learning of self-hypnosis depends on the same factors as hypnosis – responsiveness and a rapport with the person teaching it.

CHAPTER SEVEN

Manipulative and self-treatment methods for muscles and joints

Painful problems of the muscles and joints, including back pain, can usually be helped by treatment from a qualified osteopath, chiropractor or physiotherapist, who uses manipulation methods (which are becoming increasingly similar between the three disciplines) to help mobilize and normalize restricted parts of the body. Indeed, it is now accepted that chiropractic and osteopathic treatment is more effective for back and neck problems than standard medical care. Massage therapists use a wide variety of soft tissue techniques which can help muscle and ligament problems, but massage therapy differs from the work of osteopaths and chiropractors, who will have had far more training in diagnostic methods and who use joint mobilizing as well as soft tissue methods.

DIAGNOSIS BEFORE TREATMENT IS ESSENTIAL

As with any medical problem, an accurate diagnosis of what is actually causing pain is vital if treatment is to be useful and safe, and so the choice of practitioner is critical.

In the UK members of the Register of Osteopaths or College of Osteopaths can be relied on to have had a minimum of four years full-time training or six years part-time training, respectively, thereby equipping them to diagnose accurately, and to provide appropriate treatment, including rehabilitation exercises.

Members of the British Chiropractic Association will also have had four years of full-time training and will be similarly equipped to deal reliably with musculoskeletal problems. Other practitioners should be asked to give details of their training, before you decide to consult them, if they are not members of these registers. Physiotherapists will belong to the Chartered Society (MCSP) or an equivalent organization. Recently a central council has been formed in the UK to encourage higher levels of education and ethical standards in massage therapy, whilst in the USA members of the American Massage Therapy Association (AMTA) have a guaranteed standard, and they should be consulted in preference to therapists who are not members of the association.

WHAT ABOUT SEEING YOUR DOCTOR?

Few doctors of medicine have much idea of how to apply manipulative treatment for muscle and joint problems, although an increasing number are now undertaking courses to enhance their manual skills. For practical reasons, though, you may need to consult your doctor first if you have joint or back pain, but this should not necessarily stop you from also seeking advice and help from a practitioner from one or other of the professions mentioned above if reasonably rapid progress is not made in sorting out your painful musculoskeletal problem. Early osteopathic or chiropractic attention is preferable to waiting weeks or months before seeking help.

SELF-HELP METHODS

There are a number of safe and effective self-help methods derived from osteopathic and other systems which can be used as first-aid in cases of pain, strain and stiffness. If they give complete relief, then the problem was of a minor nature, but if only partial relief is experienced you should be sure to get a diagnosis and possibly professional treatment.

Strain-counterstrain methods for recent injuries and strains

In the case of recent injuries or strains and sprains (strain is an over-stretched area, while sprain is the same, but with more seriously injured tissue) apply the following simple methods and you may be amazed at the relief you get:

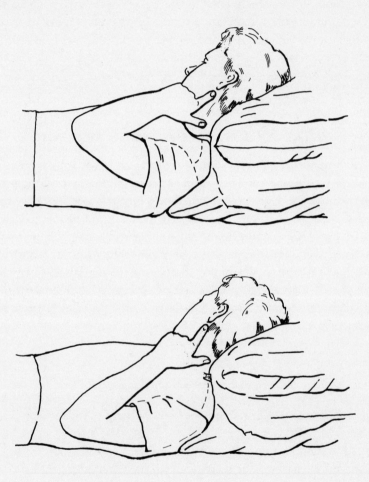

FIGURE 6 Strain-counterstrain methods enable the patient to a) *top* locate the tender spots in soft tissue such as muscle and b) *above* move the area gently to the point at which the tenderness is eased.

1. Gently test the area which causes you discomfort or pain, or which is restricted, carefully noting the direction in which particular movements cause pain. For example, it might hurt you most to turn your neck to the right and to look upwards (or restriction might be encountered), while turning left and looking down might hurt less or not at all, and be free from restriction.

2. Using this example you should search, by gentle finger or thumb pressure, for tender or 'sore' spots *in the soft tissues (muscles etc.) which would be working if the opposite movement to that which caused you pain was being performed*. In this example these would be the muscles which you use to turn your head left and look down, those on the left and front of your neck.

3. Once you have found the most tender point in these muscles keep a light pressure on it so that you can use it to guide you in the next stage of the method.

4. Now very gently and slowly move the area (in this case your head and neck) so that the tenderness goes out of the point on which you are lightly pressing. Any movement which causes you increased pain, either in the neck/head, or on that point, is in the wrong direction. You will find that there is always a position of maximum ease in which both the neck/head and the tender point will be virtually pain free. You have to find that position yourself, but there are general guidelines which tell you that if the tender point is on the front of your body you will probably have to bend forward to ease it (plus using sidebending and rotation in most cases) whereas if the tender point is on the back of your body you may have to bend backwards, along with additional 'fine-tuning' movements which may include twisting or side-bending.

   Remember that the object of your effort is to take out the tenderness from the spot on which you are pressing, but that whatever movements this calls for should not increase pain in the affected area (neck/head in this case).

5. In the example – finding it painful to turn your head right and look up – you would look in the muscles on the left and front of your neck and upper shoulder area which would be active to produce the exact opposite movement. Having found this, and holding light pressure on it, you would probably find that by letting your head tilt forward and down with a little turn to the left, and possibly sidebending to one side

or the other, while slightly lifting your left shoulder, the pain would vanish from the point. To do this you might need to be lying down so that the area is supported.

6. Once you have found the position of ease, rest there for at least a minute before slowly taking your head/neck back to a neutral position. The whole area should feel easier and less painful and restricted, and the tender point far less irritable.

7. You can do the same thing for any recent strain, sprain or restriction.

8. *What about chronic problems?* You can also use strain-counterstrain methods, exactly as described above, on any tender or sore point in any muscle in the body. If they are very chronic the relief may only be short-lived, but if recent the relief can be permanent.

It is worth re-emphasizing that strain-counterstrain will reduce pain and restriction to some extent in chronic problems, using exactly the same guidelines as for acute problems, but the results may not last very long as changes will probably have taken place in the soft tissues which would need additional treatment from a professional to normalize.

Muscle Energy Treatment (MET) for muscles and joints

There are two powerful built-in methods which you can use to safely release tight and tense muscles, often a cause of continuing pain and stiffness. These are post isometric relaxation (PIR) and reciprocal inhibition (RI).

PIR: When a muscle has been contracted for seven seconds or more without being allowed to move (known as an isometric exercise or contraction) it will be far more pliable and easy to stretch after the contraction than before it. This effect is physiologically normal, and we can use it to help to free and stretch tight painful tissues very gently.

RI: When a muscle is contracted isometrically it causes its opposing muscle to relax, allowing it to be stretched more easily and painlessly after the contraction. The muscle which opposes another is known as its antagonist. Every muscle has antagonists, or we would only be able to move ourselves in one direction and not back again.

If the muscles which turn your head to the right are tense and painful,

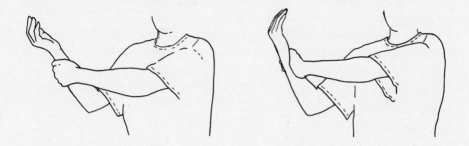

FIGURE 7 In a) *left* the left arm provides resistance while the patient attempts to straighten the right arm; this form of isometric contraction is using reciprocal inhibition (RI), which would in this case leave the upper arm more relaxed. Post-isometric relaxation (PIR) is another method of producing the same result: b) *right* shows the patient attempting to *bend* her right arm against resistance from her left.

try to turn your head to the left against resistance from your hand pressure (to do this sit at a table with your head resting in your hands). As you turn your head to the left you will be contracting the muscles which might be tight, stopping easy movement to the right. After a ten second contraction, using only about 20 per cent of your strength, resisted by your own hands, you should – because of PIR – be able to more easily and painlessly turn your head to the right. The muscles on the left will have been forced to relax painlessly.

Or, you could use RI as you try resisting your attempt to actually turn your head to the right (as long as the effort is not painful) and this would use the antagonists of the muscles which are probably short (on the left side) and which are preventing easy movement to the right. After the contraction is over (ten seconds or so) there would have been inhibition of the muscles on the left and it should be more easy to turn to the right. Even if you have no obvious problem, try this method. Sit at a table resting your head in your hands as you try to release tightness in your neck muscles to increase the range of rotation (we all have enough tension to demonstrate the improvement these simple methods can produce).

- Never apply more than about 20 per cent of the strength in muscles when using RI or PIR.
- Never cause pain when doing these exercises. If you do you are either

using too much effort or should switch to antagonist muscles, as the ones you are using are too sensitive.

- After the contraction wait a few seconds until you have relaxed, and then gently stretch the tissues (muscles etc.) a little further than they could go before the contraction. Repeat the exercise as often as you like, as long as no pain is caused, and you will gain extra amounts of stretch each time.
- You will get better results from PIR than from RI, but may have to use RI if PIR proves painful.

You can use Muscle Energy methods on any stiffness or painful area to release tension in the muscles whether the restriction/stiffness is a muscle or a joint. Even an arthritic joint can be made more flexible, if only for a short time, by this treatment as long as you stick precisely to the guidelines given above.

When should you choose counterstrain and when MET?

Counterstrain is best for acute problems, and is ideal if there is muscle spasm associated with it (lumbago and wry neck are two good examples). MET is best for restrictions, stiffness and limited range of movement, with or without painful associations. Either or both can be used on any given pain/stiffness problem, one to ease spasm and pain and the other to increase range of movement.

Note: Self-treatment using these methods should not replace professional advice unless complete relief is achieved after using them just once or twice. They are ideal methods for first-aid and to support what is being done by skilled health care professionals.

Dealing with trigger points for pain relief

Many people suffer years of pain, for example chronic headaches, which have nothing to do with the area in which they feel the pain because it is, in fact, being exported there from somewhere else, from a trigger point. As I explained earlier in the book, certain muscular areas of the body can become 'facilitated' (extremely easily irritated) because of mechanical and other forms of stress. When this happens the nerve impulses which pass through, or which derive from them, become increasingly sensitive and capable of causing quite severe pain in distant 'target' areas.

Examples of common triggers and targets include head pain which comes from triggers in the neck and shoulder muscles; abdominal pain which comes from triggers in the back; breast pain which comes from arm muscle triggers; knee pain which comes from triggers in the thigh and foot; and toe pain which comes from triggers in the shin area.

There are many more such patterns (see below) which can be successfully treated using either pain killing injections, acupuncture, acupressure, chilling techniques (cryotherapy), soft tissue manipulation techniques, electrotherapy or other methods, some of which (mainly pressure and stretch techniques) can be self-applied. Injection and acupuncture should be professionally administered.

When should you suspect that your pain is from trigger points? If your pain has no obvious cause, such as a joint strain, an arthritic condition etc., and seems persistent despite treatment or rest, or after you have had treatment for a problem which was supposed to be the cause, you might start suspecting trigger point activity.

Be especially suspicious of trigger point activity if your pain is worse when different forms of stress are current, say after physical effort, or emotional upset, or a chill, or any other form of stress, whether or not it directly involves the area of pain.

How to find trigger points

- If you carefully search with your fingers through muscles which are sensitive or tight you will find very tender local areas of muscle which seem more fibrous, stringy or even slightly swollen, which when you press them (for three to four seconds) cause a new pain to appear some distance away. The new pain is in what is called a target area, and this might well be a place where you have been feeling pain for some time.
- If you have a recurrent ache or pain in a part of your body (head, face, back, hips etc.) which does not seem to be worse when you press carefully with your fingers on the area, or which seems to have no obvious cause, then use the trigger point maps and information to see whether these might not themselves be target areas, by working backwards from the target to where the trigger is usually found for pain in that place. Press into this area with a finger or thumb, and see if you

can reproduce the pain in the target area. If you can you have found the trigger point, and you will need to treat it or have it treated professionally by a suitable therapist.

What to do to triggers when you find them
Many ways exist for successfully treating trigger points yourself.

(a) The point needs to be deactivated to some extent, and you can do this by using direct finger, thumb or tennis ball pressure in the following way. First use enough pressure so that you can just feel the pain in the target area and hold this pressure for about seven to ten seconds before easing off, not letting go of the place, but not applying any pressure for a further five seconds. Repeat this process of ten seconds or so of pressure followed by five seconds of rest for up to two minutes (no more than eight full cycles of on and off pressure.) Or, stop just as soon as the referred (target area) pain feels that it is lessening.

(b) Instead of this pressure method you can try to start deactivating the trigger point by using the counterstrain method described earlier in this chapter. After either two minutes of pressure or at least a minute of 'ease' in the appropriate counterstrain position you will need to move to the next stage of the self-treatment.

(c) The next stage is to stretch the muscles in which the trigger point is sited, and you can try using MET to do this if the muscle is in a suitable place; it is very hard to stretch muscles between your shoulder blades yourself but quite easy to stretch those between your neck and shoulder (a common trigger point area). Unfortunately, unless the muscles in which trigger points lie are stretched after treatment the trigger will very soon become active again. *So, stretching is a must.* Ideally you should be having the treatment done by a skilled therapist, but if this is not possible, follow the guidelines given below.

(d) It is preferable, during the stretching, for the muscle in which the trigger point lies to be chilled. One good way of doing this is to roll over the muscle (for no more than about 20 seconds in any one minute) a can which has been in a freezer, using slow sweeps from the trigger point towards the target area. An easy way of doing this is to fill an empty soft drink can with water and freeze it. (See also 'ice massage' on page 101)

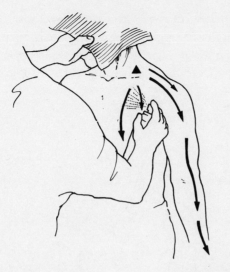

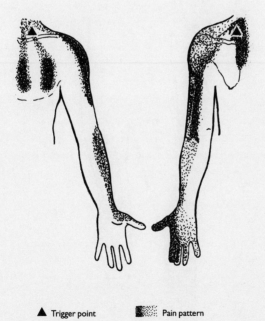

▲ Trigger point   ▓ Pain pattern

FIGURE 8 The Stretch/Chill method involves stretching and then chilling the affected muscle. This example illustrates treatment of the scaleni muscles: a) *top* shows the patient's face being shielded from an ice-cold spray, applied at the trigger point and in sweeping movements towards the target (painful) areas, as shown in b) *above*.

(e) After treating the trigger point, rest the whole area for a day or so, avoiding any strenuous movements. Immediately after the treatment placing a damp, hot towel (rung out in hot water) over the previously treated point for 15 minutes is helpful and soothing.

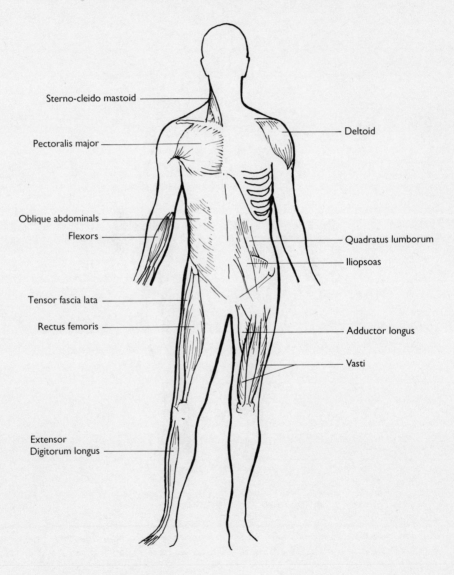

FIGURE 9 Postural or endurance muscles.

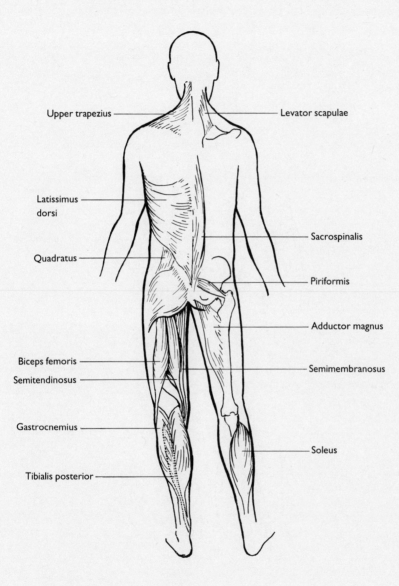

Upper trapezius

Levator scapulae

Latissimus
dorsi

Sacrospinalis

Quadratus

Piriformis

Adductor magnus

Biceps femoris

Semimembranosus

Semitendinosus

Gastrocnemius

Soleus

Tibialis posterior

FIGURE 10 Postural or endurance muscles.

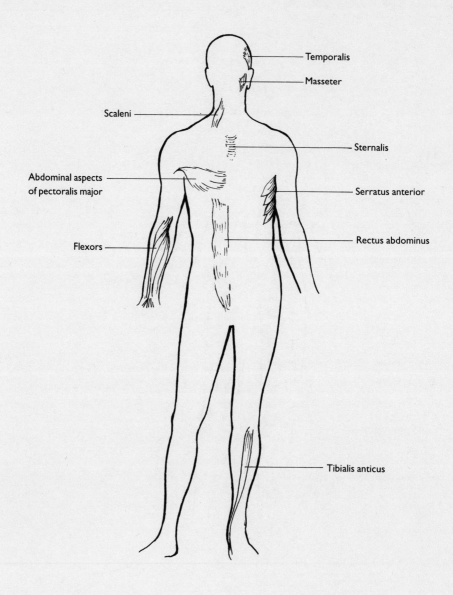

FIGURE II Phasic muscles.

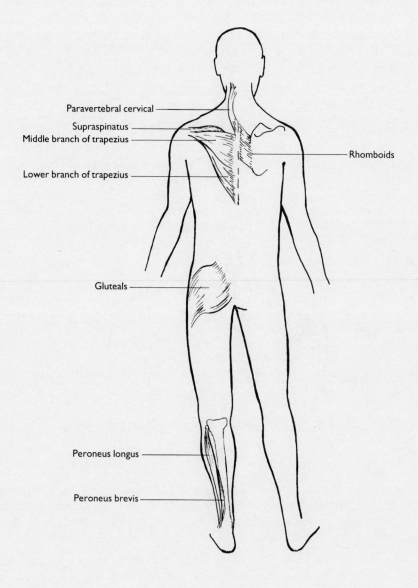

FIGURE 12 Phasic muscles.

Some of the main trigger/target patterns

1. Triggers found along the upper surface and top/inner angle of shoulder blade triggers refer pain to the head, face, neck and shoulders.
2. The border of the shoulder blade near the spine or its lower angle refers to target areas in the upper arms and to the little finger side of the hand; sometimes to the front of the shoulders.
3. Triggers in the *upper trapezius* (running from the base of the skull to the shoulder) refer pain to the area behind the ear or the forehead. Search this muscle by gentle squeezing/pinching rather than pressure.

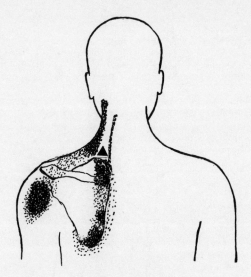

FIGURE 13 The levator scapulae trigger and target areas.

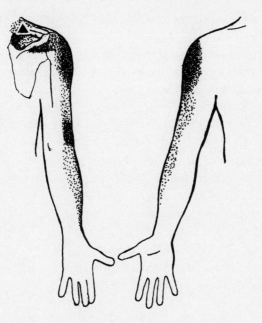

FIGURE 14 The supraspinatus trigger and target areas.

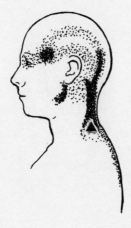

FIGURE 15 The upper trapezius trigger and target areas.

4. Triggers on the upper surface of the sacral bone (base of spine) are involved in many pain problems.

5. Low back pain is also associated with triggers on the outer border of the large muscles near the spine at waist level (*quadratus lumborum*). Pressure to reach triggers here needs to be from the side of the muscle not from the back.

6. Sometimes pressure here accesses triggers in the *latissimus dorsi* muscle which will refer pain to the shoulder or arm.

7. The muscles of the buttock (*glutei*) carry triggers, especially just under the rim of the pelvic bones, which can send pain to the hips, down the leg (back usually) and outer foot.

8. Pain down the leg which mimics sciatic pain is also caused by triggers in the *piriformis* muscle which can lie just behind the hip joint or a little further back towards the *sacrum*.

9. Trigger points lying on the back of the leg, about four inches above the knee, refer pain of the knee and calf.

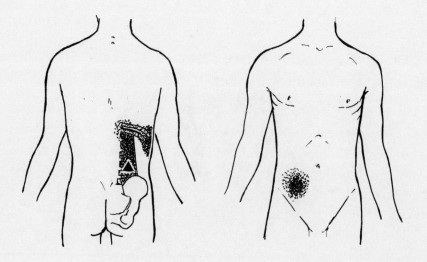

FIGURE 16 The quadratus lumborum trigger and target areas.

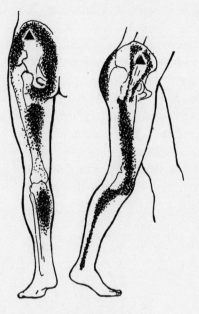

FIGURE 17 The gluteus minimus trigger and target areas.

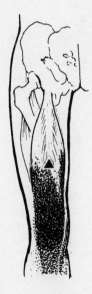

FIGURE 18 The biceps femoris (hamstring) trigger and target areas.

10. Lower calf pain can also result from a trigger which lies just below the broadest part of the calf in the *gastrocnemius* muscle, or lower in the calf in the *soleus* muscle.

11. Triggers in the neck muscles can refer to the shoulders or the head/face.

12. Search for triggers by gentle squeezing of the *sternomastoid* muscle working up towards the mastoid bone (behind the ear) from the lower part of the muscle where it inserts into the collar bone (central and mid-line part) and the upper surface of the breastbone. Triggers refer pain to the face and head.

13. In the same area of the side/front of the neck lie the *scalene* muscles which house triggers which refer to the arm and hand.

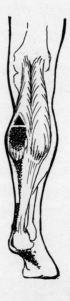

FIGURE 19 The gastrocnemius trigger and target areas.

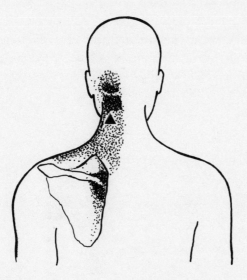

FIGURE 20 The posterior cervical trigger and target areas.

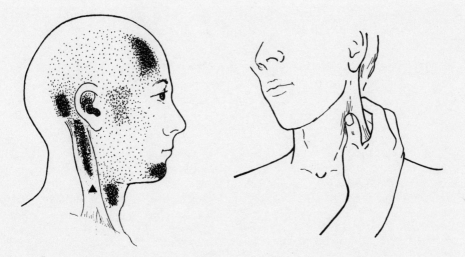

FIGURE 21 a) *left* the sternomastoid trigger and target areas. b) *right* A squeezing technique, applied here to the sternomastoid muscles (and scaleni, see Figure 8 b), can help to locate pain trigger points.

14. Triggers which are found in the jaw muscles refer to the tempero-mandibular joint and can be a cause of tinnitus and eye problems.
15. Triggers in the *pectoral* muscles and just below the collar bone can refer to the arm, or into the chest, or down the side of the body.
16. Triggers which lie in the small muscles between the ribs can refer to the chest, back or internal regions.

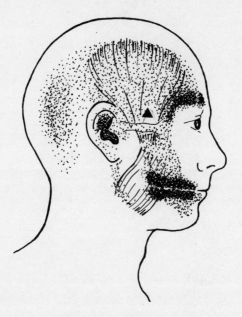

FIGURE 22 The temporalis and masseter trigger and target areas.

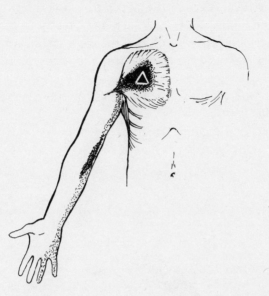

FIGURE 23 The pectoralis major (clavicular division) trigger and target areas.

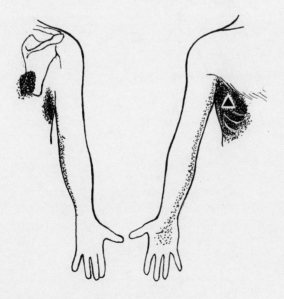

FIGURE 24 The serratus anterior trigger and target areas.

17. The large *biceps* muscle in the upper arm inserts into the arm by a tendon, and in this area triggers are found which refer to the shoulder.
18. On the breastbone (sternum) itself there is very little muscle, and yet triggers can be found which refer across the chest to either shoulder or both.
19. Abdominal muscle triggers can refer to the sides, downwards or up towards the chest.
20. Trigger points on the inner thigh refer to the hip, or down the leg to the knee.

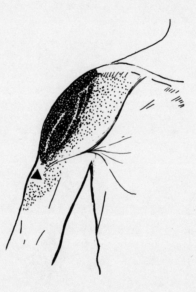

FIGURE 25 The deltoid (biceps) trigger and target areas.

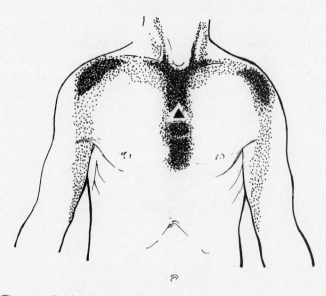

FIGURE 26 The sternalis trigger and target areas.

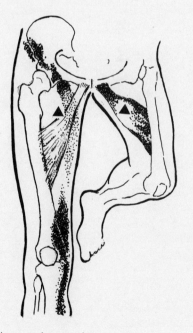

FIGURE 27 The adductor longus trigger and target areas.

21. Triggers in the muscles of the side of the thigh (*tensor fascia lata*) produce sciatic type pain.
22. Triggers in the front of the lower leg refer to the foot and ankle.

Note: These examples represent the major triggers. There are hundreds of others which can exist.

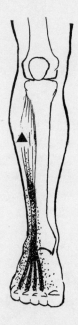

FIGURE 28 The extensor digitorum longus trigger and target areas.

Self-massage for pain relief

Two key features help maintain pain when muscles are tense and tight, inadequate supply of fresh oxygenated blood and retention/congestion/build-up of waste products in the tissues. Massage can very successfully help normalize both these features, even if this is only for a short time. Massage also produces relaxation and reduction in anxiety levels (especially when skilfully performed) and to some extent self-massage can achieve this too. Self-massage involves application of rhythmic strokes to the muscles in a systematic manner.

Caution

Do not give yourself or anyone else a massage, unless you have professional approval or instruction, in the following circumstances:

- On tissues which are actively inflamed or where blood vessels are inflamed.
- Where active infection is present.
- If there is a heart condition.
- If there is a cancerous condition.
- If there has been haemorrhage or other causes of bleeding in the tissues.
- In the area of a recent fracture or sprain.

Basic techniques

The following techniques are easily learned. Massage should never hurt, and should be performed slowly and rhythmically.

EFFLEURAGE

A massage cream or oil should be applied gently to the skin over the area to be massaged so that no drag occurs on the skin. At first long, slow strokes are called for, using the heels of the hands, the palms of the hands or the thumbs. Your hands should be relaxed but firm and should mould themselves to the shape and contours of the area being worked on. No pain should be produced and the pressure should match the sensitivity of the area.

Ideally, as one hand is moving forwards over the area, the other should be coming back so that an alternating, rhythmic series of pleasant stroking

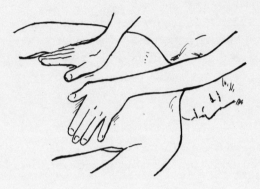

FIGURE 29 Effleurage is a form of massage employing alternating rhythmic strokes.

actions soothes the region. Often a circular action is appropriate so that one hand is following the other in slow circles.

On a large area such as the thigh, make a stroke away from you with the heel of your hand for about 12 inches (30 cm), and then circle back again. As your hand is slowly returning towards you, the other begins its stroke. You are now doing effleurage.

Continue with this sort of approach for several minutes, varying the area slightly after a few repetitions. Use a similar pattern again after some of the other methods described below, and perhaps finish the whole session with stroking as well.

PETRISSAGE

This action is a kneading, wringing one in which muscles are held and lifted by one hand and then the other. One hand grasps a handful of muscle firmly but gently, lifting and pulling it towards you while the other pushes the adjacent tissue away from you, producing a kneading, squeezing and wringing action.

Start by pressing downwards with the heel of one hand while you lift

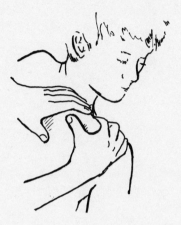

FIGURE 30 Petrissage involves a kneading, wringing action.

the tissue with the fingers and thumb of that hand. With a handful of muscle, lift and gently squeeze or roll it before letting the other hand take over the same task. Repeat this process of one hand releasing its grip as the other takes over (just like making bread) rhythmically several times before moving to another part of the muscle. In some areas two hands can lift simultaneously lifting, wringing and twisting the tissues.

TAPPING
Tapping and vibration of tissues can be very relaxing and can reduce pain sensations markedly. Try shaking the tissues gently, getting a vibration effect or with the side of the hand make a series of chopping actions towards the muscle so that the finger tips (relaxed) strike the muscle like drumsticks hitting a drum. By doing this quickly and repetitively a very pleasing sensation can be created.

THUMB WORK
Wherever you feel local tension in the muscles or bands of tight tense tissues, use your thumbs or the heels of your hands to push across or into

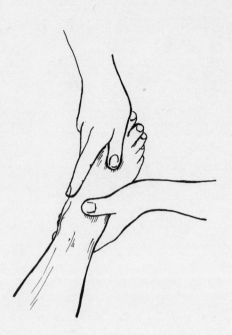

FIGURE 31 Firm pressure from the thumbs can be used to release tension in muscles or bands of tissue.

the area, never to cause pain but sufficiently hard to produce a 'nice hurt'. Hold such pressure for up to ten seconds at a time before moving on or applying a gentle effleurage to sooth it.

TENNIS BALL MASSAGE

Some areas are hard to reach, such as the low back, and you may need help to massage here. Place a tennis ball on the carpet and lie onto it so that it presses in the area of muscular pain. Gently roll over it so that it presses and pushes the muscle until you feel easier; or tie two tennis balls into a sock so that they lie together with a small space between. Lie on this so that the balls are on each side of the spine, and roll gently up and down to 'release' tight muscles. A similar effect can be achieved for the sole of the foot using a squash ball.

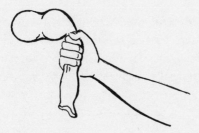

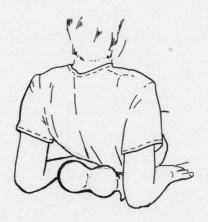

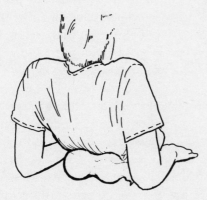

FIGURE 32 Tennis ball massage is ideal for areas that are hard to reach, such as those to the sides of the spine.

Exercise for pain relief

Well-chosen exercises can be very helpful in rehabilitation programmes where pain is a feature of musculoskeletal problems. It is essential to ensure that exercises do not make matters worse. Ideally, therefore, an exercise programme should be chosen and taught by a skilled health professional. Because of the very individual nature of exercise and rehabilitation programmes it is almost impossible to give guidelines except of a most general type.

- Stretching (yoga or muscle-energy type) and movement in water are the safest forms of movement therapy. Fast repetitive exercises/movements are more likely to be irritating to pain conditions than slowly performed stretching.
- In any given painful condition, if you move the area or other parts of the body very carefully in all possible directions, some will be more and some less painful than the others. You can use MET (PIR and RI) methods to increase your pain-free range before doing such an assessment. If you can identify which movements cause no increase in pain at the time they are performed *or afterwards* you can begin to build up a sequence of simple exercises (in water or at home) which will help maintain muscle tone and circulation. For example, you may find that it is painless to move your arm in one or two directions, but painful to move it in others. Slowly take it in the painless directions a number of times, several times daily, in order to keep muscles toned and circulation active. If actual movement is too painful, just tensing and relaxing the various muscles of the area can do a lot of good as well. After doing whatever pain-free exercises you can several times a day (never allowing them to increase pain levels) you can retest the direction and range of pain-free motion after a week or so, and introduce any new pain-free movements which may have developed.
- If the area of pain is too great to allow it to be moved, then see whether movements of areas distant to it will allow you to help circulation and muscle tone (for example, if your low back is too painful to move in any direction, then arm and leg movements which don't hurt the back can be useful).
- There is evidence aplenty that thinking about a particular movement

slightly activates the muscles which would perform that action, so it even helps just to visualize particular movements, even if they cannot be performed because of pain.

- Similarly, eye movements activate muscles in the direction in which the eyes are moving. If you look upwards, for example, without moving your neck and head, the muscles which bend your neck and back backwards will increase in tone in preparation for that movement.
- Aerobic exercises are possible if they don't increase pain or irritate existing conditions (take advice on this). It is well established that such activity reduces stress levels, reduces anxiety and produces some release of natural pain-killing substances by the body.
- If there are any joint problems – ankles, knees, hips or back – introduce cushioned innersoles or use well padded trainers. The reduction in 'shock' which this simple adaptation can create is quite astounding; reducing the degree of stress in weight-bearing joints by up to a half.

Vibration therapy

In the American Civil War the pain in amputation stumps was commonly treated with a very successful form of vibration, but it was not until the mid-1940s that this was revived and used in modern medicine. Pain relief achieved in this way often lasts for hours, and sometimes days. It is ideal for chronic pain, but not much use in acute conditions. Research amongst amputees in the USA has shown it to be frequently more effective than the use of TENS. The only drawback is finding an appropriate vibrator. The best are small battery operated vibration units available from most pharmacies. These are cheap to buy and easy to use. Best results are obtained from using a high frequency – between 100 and 200 Hz.

The advantage of TENS is that it is unobtrusive and can be worn with no-one knowing, and can therefore be used in any setting. A vibrator can really only be used in private.

Vibration from a 100 Hz machine should be applied near or below the painful site with a moderate amount of pressure, and this should be maintained for *at least 45 minutes*. If a machine with a lower frequency is used, or if only light pressure is applied and for a shorter time, then the results will be less good.

The pain-reducing effect is known as hyperstimulation analgesia. It does not result from the release of endorphins, but from the vibration sensations passing along large fibres and blocking or reducing access by pain sensations – the 'gate' theory in action. Ideally, vibration therapy should be reserved for chronic pain which proves unresponsive to the other methods described in this chapter.

CHAPTER EIGHT

Hydrotherapy

Hydrotherapy can be effectively applied at home, and it puts at your disposal a number of simple and efficient ways to alleviate pain problems. Here are some of them:

- Cold applications can help to reduce the sensitivity of painful nerve endings.
- The inflammation which often accompanies pain can be lessened.
- Hot and cold compress techniques can reduce the congestion or swelling which often results in stiffness and discomfort.
- Long cold applications can reduce the speed of blood flow to an area, thus reducing the chance of bruising.
- Contrast bathing, involving 'warming' compresses, cold douches, hot and cold applications etc., can help when sluggish circulation resulting from inactivity or muscle tension has led to poor tissue oxygenation and consequent pain.
- Hydrotherapy's 'warming' compresses (they go on cold but warm up from body heat) and alternating hot and cold applications or immersions can relax muscles and ease stiffness.
- Pain such as that generated by trigger points or inflammation can be eased by use of ice or alternating hot and cold applications.
- General anxiety, which increases pain perception, can be helped enormously by the use of a neutral bath or wet sheet pack.
- There are many ways of using different substances in water to assist in

pain relief, including Epsom salts and a range of essential oils.

- Steam, with or without the addition of aromatic herbs/oils, can be used to reduce the pain of chest and sinus congestion.

Overall, cold is more helpful than heat when correctly applied to injuries and inflamed areas, and hot hydrotherapy methods should almost always end with a short cold application. There follows a list of ground rules to adhere to when using hydrotherapy:

- Hot applications result in dilation (opening up) of local tissues, followed by adjacent blood vessels importing additional blood. Relaxation of muscles follows application of heat.
- Short cold applications at first contract blood vessels, reducing circulation and decongesting tissues. This is followed by a reaction in which blood vessels open and tissues are flushed with fresh oxygen-rich blood.
- Alternation of heat and cold produces circulatory interchange and increased drainage and oxygenation of tissues.
- As a general rule, unless otherwise stated, there should always be a short cold application or immersion after a hot one (and preferably also before).
- When heat is applied in hydrotherapy it should not be so hot that it scalds the skin. It should always be bearable in intensity.
- The general rules of hot and cold applications tell us that:
  Short cold applications stimulate circulation.
  Long cold applications (less than a minute) depress circulation and metabolism.
  Long hot applications leave the area congested and static, and demand a cold application to help restore normality.
  Short hot applications (less than five minutes) stimulate circulation, but long hot (longer than five minutes) applications depress both circulation and metabolism drastically.
- In hydrotherapy, temperatures are defined as follows:

Hot:	98–104 deg F	(36–40 deg C)
Neutral/Warm:	93–97 deg F	(34–36 deg C)
Tepid:	81–92 deg F	(26–33 deg C)
Cool:	66–80 deg F	(18–26 deg C)
Cold:	55–65 deg F	(12–18 deg C)

Reflex effects can be used since certain parts of the body, when heated or cooled, will have reflex effects on the circulation of distant areas.

- People with poor circulation or low vitality should not be subjected to extremes of temperature. It is better in such cases to use a contrast of warm to cool rather than hot to cold.
- Avoid treating with hydrotherapy soon after a meal. Leave it for at least an hour and a half.
- Diabetics should avoid *any* heat treatments to their legs.

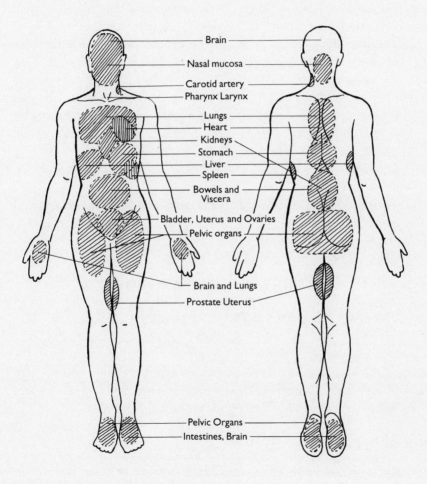

Brain
Nasal mucosa
Carotid artery
Pharynx Larynx
Lungs
Heart
Kidneys
Stomach
Liver
Spleen
Bowels and Viscera
Bladder, Uterus and Ovaries
Pelvic organs
Brain and Lungs
Prostate Uterus
Pelvic Organs
Intestines, Brain

FIGURE 33 The major hydro-reflex connections.

- Do not use hydrotherapy in circumstances of:
    extremely fragile skin;
    skin conditions which are irritated by moisture;
    areas of numbness;
    serious circulatory conditions.
- The main *reflex* connections are:
    The skin of the feet and hands with the circulation of the head, chest and pelvic regions (especially bladder and reproductive organs, including prostate in men).
    The skin of the lower breast bone and the kidneys.
    The skin of the face with the blood vessels of the head.
    The skin of the base of the neck area is reflexively connected with the nasal mucosa (which is why cold on the back of the neck stops a nose-bleed).
    The skin overlying various spinal regions connects with the internal organs supplied by nerves from that spinal level (lungs and heart with upper thoracic spine; stomach and liver with middle thoracic spine; bowels and abdominal organs with lower back).
    The skin of the thighs, low back and buttocks relates to genito-urinary organs.
    The skin of the lower/inner thighs connects with the prostate and uterus.

HYDROTHERAPY METHODS

Heating compress (called 'cold compress' in Europe)

Treatment suggestion
Any painful joint, mastitis, sore throat (compress on throat from ear to ear and supported over top of head), backache (ideally compress should cover abdomen and back), sore tight chest from bronchitis.

Materials required

- A single or double sheet of cotton large enough to cover the area to be treated (double for people with good circulation/vitality, single for

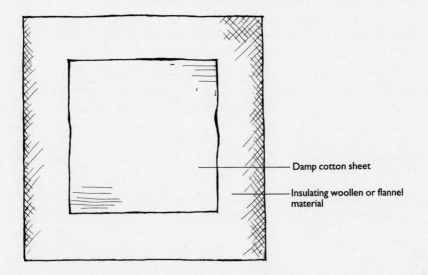

FIGURE 34 A heating compress (also known as a cold compress).

people with only moderate circulation/vitality).
- One thickness of woollen or flannel material larger than the cotton material so that it can cover it completely with no edges protruding.
- Plastic material of same size as woollen material.
- Safety pins.
- Cold water.

Method
Ring out cotton material in cold water so that it is damp but not dripping wet. Place this over painful area and immediately cover with woollen/flannel material (and also the plastic material if there is good robust vitality) and safety pin snugly in place. The compress should be firm enough so that no air can get in to cool it, but not so tight that circulation is restricted. The cold material will rapidly warm up and feel comfortable. After several hours it should be virtually dry.

Use the warming compress up to four times daily, with at least an hour between applications. Ideally leave it on overnight.

Wash the material used before reusing as it will have absorbed acid wastes from the body.

Caution: If for any reason (too wet, too loose, poor vitality) the compress is still cold after 20 minutes, then remove it and give the area a brisk rub with a towel.

Note:

At times an application of a cold damp cloth to an area is called for (perhaps after addition of a soothing substance such as arnica extract) to a recently injured area (e.g. 'black eye'). This is a true *'cold' compress* and will be referred to as such, whereas the compress which goes on cold and becomes warm (as above) will be given its more accurate American name of a *warming or heating compress*.

Fomentations

Treatment suggestion

Pain and congestion especially involving muscle spasm and tension; lumbago and neuralgia between the ribs; dysmenorrhoea; kidney stones (renal colic).

Not to be used in:

All cases of cancer; heart disease; diabetes mellitus; circulatory problems in the legs; haemorrhage; sensitive skin.

Materials required

Sheet, blanket, towels, very hot water, woollen material for fomentation (towel will do, but is less efficient), bowl with hot water and mustard.

Method

(Note: This treatment is impossible to do for yourself, so someone has to help with the applications.)

Sit in an upright chair with your feet in a bowl of bearably hot water (104 degrees Fahrenheit/40 degrees Celsius) in which two or three teaspoonsful of mustard powder have been dissolved.

Uncover the area to be treated and have a sheet and blanket handy to cover this and as much of the body as possible once the fomentation has been applied.

Wring out woollen or towelling fomentation material in very hot water (the more water retained the more effective the fomentation) and place immediately between dry larger towels (several layers).

Apply insulated hot towels to the painful area and cover immediately with sheet and blanket. If it is too hot for comfort, remove for a few seconds, drying the skin, then replace.

Change to a new fomentation application every five minutes but between each application place a cold wet towel on the area for about five to ten seconds.

After the second fomentation application, or when sweating begins, apply a cold towel to the forehead.

Repeat the application of hot fomentations a total of three or four times. After the last fomentation is removed, use a damp, cold towel to briskly friction rub the area and the body as a whole (not for dysmenorrhoea), and then rest in a warm and comfortable position for half an hour to an hour.

This can be done daily, if helpful, but the skin should be protected with Vaseline (or similar) if repeated frequently. The heat of fomentations promotes sweating and elimination of toxic wastes, relaxes local spasm and reduces pain.

Neutral bath

Treatment suggestion
This is a superb relaxation method, reducing anxiety and relieving chronic pain.

Not to be used in:
Skin conditions which react badly to water, or if there is serious cardiac disease (it can be helpful, but get professional advice first).

Materials required
A bathtub and a bath thermometer.

Method
Run a bath as full as possible and with the water as close to 97 degrees Fahrenheit (36 degrees Celsius) as possible, and certainly not exceeding

that temperature. The bath has its effect by being as close to body temperature as possible. Immersion in water at this neutral temperature has a profoundly relaxing, sedating effect and a calming influence on nervous system activity.

Get into the bath so that if possible the water covers your shoulders, and support your head on a towel or sponge.

The thermometer should be in the bath, and the temperature of the water should not be allowed to drop below 92 degrees Fahrenheit (33 degrees Celsius). It can be topped up periodically, but the temperature must not exceed the limit specified above. The duration of the bath can be anything from 30 minutes to four hours. The longer the better as far as relaxation effects are concerned.

After the bath, pat dry quickly and get into bed for at least an hour.

Full sheet pack

Treatment suggestion
The full sheet pack has the remarkable effect of passing through four distinct stages of activity each of which has different influences on the person receiving it and each stage has different indications. Described simply these are:

- An initial cooling stage indicated for feelings of general weakness or if there is a fever.
- A neutral stage (when the pack is the same temperature as the body) which has the same indications as a neutral bath, especially agitation, anxiety and nervousness.
- A hot stage which helps in a number of health conditions, but from the pain perspective is most useful if there is sinus congestion/pain, bowel discomfort (especially if constipated) or conditions such as colitis involving the colon.
- A stage when sweating becomes profuse which is used for detoxification from drugs (including tobacco), alcohol or during some infections to speed up rash development.

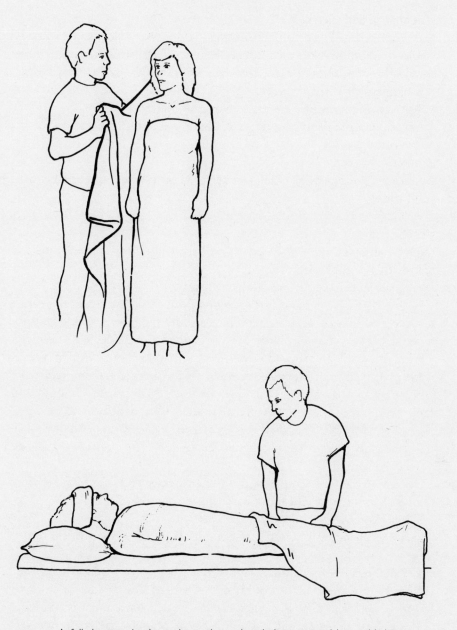

FIGURE 35 A full sheet pack: a) *top* shows the patient being wrapped in a cold damp sheet and then a dry sheet before b) *above* lying on a blanket which is wrapped around the body so that the sheets are entirely covered.

Not to be used in:
Avoid stages three and four if anaemic or very weak/debilitated. Being wrapped, mummy-like, can induce feelings of claustrophobia so there should always be someone handy to help with removal of the pack in case this happens or you feel unwell.

Skin conditions which are made worse by water.

Anyone with diabetes should take advice before using a wet pack.

Materials required
Two cotton sheets; two woollen blankets; towels; pillow; hot water bottle; hand towel.

Method
(Note: This treatment is impossible to do for yourself, so someone has to help with the application.)

Place a blanket on the bed and open fully.

Have a warm shower and, on emerging from this, have someone ready to wrap you in a cold wet sheet which should have been wrung out in water at between 60 and 70 degrees Fahrenheit (15–21 degrees Celsius).

Working swiftly, this should be wrapped from under your armpits so that it fits snugly to your body right down to the ankles, and immediately covered by second sheet (dry) before you lie on the blanket which should then be wrapped around you from neck to feet, with no sheet being allowed to be visible (thus denying access to air which would keep it cool).

The second blanket should be placed over the first one and tucked around you snugly.

Use towels and/or neck pillow to insulate areas such as the neck, where the blanket may not efficiently be enclosing the pack.

Place a hot water bottle near your feet.

Speed of operation is essential as chilling will occur if the work is done slowly.

When the third and fourth stages are reached a cold compress to the forehead is a good idea, as would be the offer of sips of water if thirsty. Sweating can be profuse in stage four, so water replenishment is needed.

The pack can be discontinued at or after any of the four stages as appropriate. For full benefit it should run its course, which takes up to three hours or more depending upon your vitality (how much heat you generate).

If at any time after the first few minutes the pack feels uncomfortably cold it should be stopped and a brisk friction rub applied to stimulate circulation. The coldness would indicate either that the sheet was too wet or the water too cold, or that the insulation was inadequately applied.

Ice pack and ice massage

Treatment suggestion
All sprains and injuries; bursitis and other joint swellings/inflammations (unless cold aggravates the pain); toothache and headache; haemorrhoids; bites.

Not to be used in:
Avoid abdominal applications during acute bladder problems; over chest with acute asthma; if condition is aggravated by cold.

Materials required
A piece of flannel (wool) material large enough to cover area to be treated; towels; ice; safety pins; plastic sheet; bandage.

Method
Place crushed ice to a thickness of an inch or so onto the towel, and fold and pin it to contain the ice. Place the flannel onto the site of pain and put the ice pack onto this.

Cover pack with plastic sheet and use bandage to hold the whole thing in place.

Protect clothing/bedding with additional plastic sheets/towels.

Leave in place for up to half an hour, and repeat after an hour if helpful.

For ice massage
Use either ice (messy as it melts) or something metallic which has been in a freezer, such as a soft-drink can which has been emptied of its original contents, filled with water and frozen. Seal the hole and use this to roll over the painful area to chill it, while ensuring that the skin does not frost or become irritated. Several minutes of slowly moving iced metal over a joint or painful area will relieve a good deal of pain. If at the same time

gentle stretching or painless movement can be introduced the benefits are enhanced.

Or apply a cold spray as used on acute sporting injuries. Take care with these as they can blanch and damage skin, although if used in slow sweeps they are very useful.

Poultices (including charcoal, clay, herbal or vegetable)

Treatment suggestion
Painful congested or inflamed areas; insect bites and stings; to bring boils and abscesses to a head; counter-irritant in painful swellings.

Not to be used in:
Avoid use if boil or abscess is open and pustular, as poultice can encourage bacterial activity once site has opened. Avoid any substance to which the patient may be allergic.

Materials required
Sufficient quantity of the chosen substance which should have been reduced to a pulp or paste by mixing with water or by shredding or pulverizing. These can include charcoal; French green clay or bentonite; shredded or pulped cabbage, potato or carrot or specific herbs (such as hops, flax/linseed, comfrey); hot water; cloth (cotton for preference) large enough to hold the pulp/paste and cover the treated area; plastic sheet to cover this and prevent leakage; woollen material large enough to cover the plastic sheet; safety pin or bandage; towels.

Method
Ensure that the chosen material (see below) is in paste or pulp form by mixing powders (mustard, charcoal, clay) with hot water or by shredding/pulverizing the herb or vegetable. If possible, the material should be hot on application, although this will not apply to vegetable/herb poultices which will warm by absorption of body heat.

Place paste directly onto skin or onto cotton material which is then placed so that the material is in contact with the skin.

Once the material is on the skin, cover the cotton with the plastic sheet, and then cover the plastic sheet with the wool, and pin or bandage firmly in place.

Allow to remain in skin contact for between an hour and eight hours. On removal, carefully clean skin of remaining adherent material. Cover with dry cloth.

Different materials have different benefits to offer:

POWDERED CHARCOAL

This is soothing, antiseptic and deodorant, and it absorbs vast amounts of toxic material. Ideal for joint pain/swellings, insect stings and bites.

Use up to three tablespoons of pulverized charcoal, ideally mixed with the same quantity of flax/linseed which has been reduced in a processor or seed mill. Mix with a cupful of water and bring to the boil before allowing to stand for 15 minutes. Apply to the surface of the joint or skin. This quantity will be adequate for a large joint area.

Charcoal compresses (fomentations) are a superb pain relieving method and should be used on any painful area where overlying tissues can be covered in the way described. Pain will usually diminish after five to ten minutes.

FLAXSEED/LINSEED

This seed has a gel-like consistency which makes it ideal for poultices. When used alone it has a soothing and drawing quality. A tablespoon of powdered seed in a cupful of water, brought to the boil, will produce sufficient paste to cover a large joint or skin area, such as the abdomen.

CLAY/BENTONITE

The absorbent qualities of clay are enormous and make this ideal (as is charcoal) for covering open wounds and inflammatory conditions, including stings, bites, boils and carbuncles. The clay should be fine and not granular, and should be sterilized before use by baking for an hour or more in a very hot oven. Once cool, pulverize it back to a powder and mix with sufficient water to make it into a mud-like paste. Add a little (dessertspoonful) glycerine to prevent the clay sticking to the skin after use as a poultice.

HERBS AND VEGETABLE MATERIALS
Many experts believe that it is the moist, heat-retaining qualities of these which make them beneficial, rather than their particular attributes. Whether this is so, or whether there are indeed specific effects to be achieved from different plant materials used in this way waits for research to establish. Until then, availability and the ability to shred or pulp the vegetable before application are what matter most; making the potato the most practical choice.

Steam inhalation

Treatment suggestion
Painful tight chest during respiratory infections/conditions; sore throat; sinus problems.

Not to be used in:
Cardiac asthma or serious heart conditions, or anyone too frail to cope with the heat of the steam.

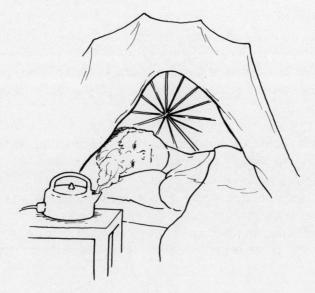

FIGURE 36 A steam inhalation with essential oils.

Materials required
Kettle and hot water; sheet; umbrella; roll of newspaper (optional); essential oils such as eucalyptus oil or wintergreen, or leaves such as mint. Aromatic herbs are optional.

Method
Bring the kettle to boil and place in a safe manner so that you can be seated close by, covered by a 'tent' made out of the umbrella and draped sheet, which also encloses the steaming kettle.

A few drops of oil, or the leaves, can be placed in the kettle, and the roll of paper placed over the spout to direct steam towards your face (this is not essential).

Breathe the steam slowly and deeply, avoiding any scalding of the skin by being too close to the spout and taking care not to upset the kettle.

Periodically use a cold damp towel to cool your face and forehead. Half an hour of stream inhalation, three times daily, helps relieve congestion.

Alternate bathing

Treatment suggestion
All painful conditions which involve congestion and inflammation, locally or generally.

Not to be used in:
Haemorrhage, colic and spasm; acute or serious chronic heart disease; acute bladder and kidney infections.

Materials required
Containers suitable for holding hot and/or cold water as well as the part to be alternatively immersed. If this is the whole pelvic area, then either large plastic or other tubs (an old-fashioned hip bath is best) are required, with a smaller container needed for simultaneous immersion of your feet; bath thermometer; hot and cold water; special ingredients (e.g. mustard).

Method
If a local area (arm, ankle etc.) is receiving treatment, then alternation of

immersion of the part into hot and cold water should follow the time guidelines given below for pelvic area in sitz baths.

For local immersion treatment ice cubes can be placed in the cold water for greater contrast. If the local area is unsuitable for such treatment by immersion (shoulder and knee could be awkward) then application to those regions of hot and cold towels soaked and lightly wrung out can be used, following the same timetable as for sitz baths given below (two to three minutes hot, followed by 30 seconds cold, at least twice, and always finish with cold).

Sitz baths are by definition the immersion of the pelvic area (buttocks and hips up to the navel) in water of one temperature, with feet in water of the same or a contrasting temperature. The sequence to follow in alternating pelvic bathing in sitz baths is:

- Two to three minutes in hot (106–110 degrees Fahrenheit/41–43 degrees Celsius)
- 30 seconds in cold (around 60 degrees F/15 degrees C)
- Two to three minutes hot
- 30 seconds cold

During the hip immersions your feet should, if possible, be in water of contrasting temperature. This may be hard to organize, in which case the alternating hip immersions alone should be used.

Note: use the timings as above for local (wrist, foot etc.) immersions, or for alternate applications of hot and cold towels to less easily immersed parts of the anatomy.

Simple bathing

This implies that no alternation of temperature occurs. An example is the *mustard bath* which is recommended in the early stages of a developing headache.

Method
One teaspoonful of powdered mustard is added to two gallons of hot water which is in a bowl large enough for both feet to rest in. A similar bowl

rests on the knees (also containing hot mustard water) into which hands and forearms are placed. Put a cool, damp cloth on your forehead.

After 20 minutes wash your hands and feet thoroughly, and rest.

Hot sitz bath

Treatment suggestion
A hot sitz bath (no alternation of hot and cold – simply pelvic immersion in hot water) is of proven value in helping speed the healing of painful anal fissures, as well as haemorrhoids, dysmenorrhoea, prostate inflammation (and bladder); pelvic inflammatory disease and atonic constipation.

Not to be used in:
Anyone with a diabetic condition.

Materials required
The same as for sitz bath, or a regular bath tub may be used.

Method
If a hip bath is available, sit in this with hot water (106–110 degrees Fahrenheit/41–43 degrees Celsius) and your feet in hot water a few degrees hotter.

If a regular bath is used, sit in it in hot water up to your navel, knees bent so that they are out of the water and feet immersed.

Apply a cold towel to your forehead during the treatment.

If anal fissures are being treated, the time spent in the bath can be up to 30 minutes. For other conditions eight minutes is adequate. At the end of the bath, rub the immersed area briefly with a towel which has been wrung out in cold water.

If prostate problems exist, hold the damp cold towel between your legs for ten seconds or so to cool the perineal area between your rectum and testicles.

Note: In some conditions, such as acute cystitis, a neutral sitz bath is useful. This involves pelvic immersion in water of neutral temperature, as in the neutral bath.

Full baths of various types

Treatment suggestion
For chronic painful conditions such as arthritis.

Not to be used in:
People with skin sensitive to whatever is being used in the bath, or who are allergic to it. Avoid Epsom salts baths if very weak and low in vitality.

Materials required
Epsom salts or a suitable essential oil, or oatmeal; bath and water.

Method
- For an Epsom salts bath dissolve 2–4 lbs in the hot water, and soak in this for 20 minutes. Briskly rub dry and get into a warm bed. Expect to perspire profusely.
- For an essential oil bath, such as chamomile (relaxing, pain relieving) use a few drops of oil suitably prepared for baths (different from that used for massage) and soak for up to half an hour.
- For an oatmeal bath (ideal for angry skin conditions such as eczema) take 1 lb (450 grams) of uncooked oatmeal and place in a gauze bag, which should be held under the hot tap as it runs, releasing the ingredients which are soothing to the skin. Float the bag in the bath while you are soaking in it and use this as a sponge to gently pat areas of irritation. The temperature of the bath water should be around 96 degrees Fahrenheit (36 degrees Celsius). Stay in this for at least 20 minutes. Pat dry afterwards. Do not rub.

WHAT ABOUT JACUZZIS OR HOT TUBS?

If you have access to a jacuzzi or hot tub this can be a help in applying heat to the painful areas of your body, along with the mechanical benefits of the underwater jets which can apply massage as well.

After any such 'treatment' always use a short cold application (such as a towel rung out in cold water) for ten seconds to the painful area or the body as a whole. A short tepid shower would do.

CHAPTER NINE

Natural medicines

Because of almost certain side-effects from most pharmaceutical drugs their use for easing chronic pain is only really justified if:

- underlying causes are being dealt with so that drug use will be short-term only;
- no cause can be found and the pain is creating serious problems for the sufferer;
- the pain is going to be self-limiting, and the treatment therefore short-term.

In these three cases the trade-off between likely side-effects and near certain benefits is acceptable. There are other options, however. These involve the use of medication which is often less toxic to our systems than proprietary synthetic drugs, or even non-toxic, and consequently more suited to long-term use.

HERBAL MEDICINE

While, traditionally, many herbal substances have been used in the treatment of pain, few have been scientifically proved to be effective. It is worth remembering, though, that aspirin is derived from a herbal extract of willow bark. Just because the practice of herbal medicine appears closer to 'nature' than the use of synthetic drugs, it does not necessarily mean that it is *always* safer to use. Indeed, some herbs are definitely toxic, especially if overused. The preference for herbal medicine rests in the fact that it has been around for a very long time and, properly prepared and properly applied, the remedies are known from experience to be relatively safe.

The warning still applies, in that the masking of pain which should be receiving attention is just as likely using herbs as it is with drugs, and it is important to remember that pain can be sending a warning message which should be listened to.

Be sure to purchase herbs and herbal medicines from reliable suppliers (your Health Food store will advise). Among the herbs which have proved their value in practice are the following:

Cayenne pepper

This contains a powerful ingredient which produces the release of a chemical involved in the pain process known as 'substance P'. Rubbing cayenne pepper extracts onto *chronically* painful areas produces a reduction in pain after an initial reddening of the area. This is usually marketed with the word 'capsicum' in the name. It is not recommended for acute pain problems.

Red chili-peppers also yield an extract (capsaicin) which can be rubbed onto painful areas such as the inflamed scars left after herpes zoster (shingles). This is available in both mild and hot versions. After an initial reddening of the area, the irritation caused by the cream and the underlying irritation of the herpes scar both tend to calm down for several days.

Chamomile

This has been shown to have marked anti-inflammatory qualities, as well as being useful in easing pain and calming spasm. It can be used internally or externally (in compresses, for example, or to bathe painful eyes) especially in cases of neuralgia, face-ache, ear-ache, and for the pain of digestive disturbance.

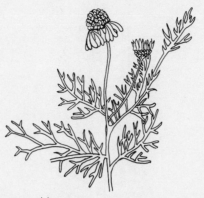

FIGURE 37 Chamomile flowers and leaves.

An ounce of the flowers boiled in a pint of water produces a large quantity of the infusion. It should be allowed to cool, and the dose is a wineglassful before each meal, and on going to bed.

Clove oil

Used for centuries for toothache, this remarkable substance is now well researched and of proven value as a pain-killer, ideally applied directly to painful dental sites, where it acts as a local anaesthetic.

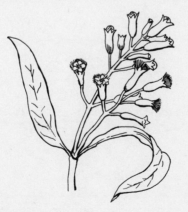

FIGURE 38 Clove flowers and fruit.

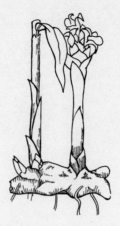

FIGURE 39 A ginger root, stem and flowers.

Ginger

Taken as a vegetable with a meal (raw/grated) or in capsule form at the end of a meal (two or three capsules) this is an excellent way of safely dealing with the discomfort of heartburn (and travel sickness as well).

Wintergreen

This has similar constituents to aspirin (salicylate) which are natural pain-killer's as well as being anti-inflammatory. Its use is recommended externally only (rub it on – don't take it by mouth).

Other herbs which have a traditional use in pain treatment, and which are safe, despite remaining in need of research, include:

Aloe vera

Extracts, or the directly gathered gel, from the leaves of this desert plant are claimed to be extremely soothing, as well as promoting healing in the treatment of burns and wounds – including frostbite, stings and bites, herpes scars and lesions, ulcers and abscesses, as well as internal conditions such as colitis, arthritis and diverticulitis.

Arnica

Used externally for recent injuries (where skin is unbroken) and for painful conditions such as frostbite or blows to the eye, where it can be added to the water of a cold compress (see Chapter 8 on Hydrotherapy).

Calendula

Used especially as an ointment for painful skin conditions, such as sunburn or injuries where the skin has been broken.

Echinacea (purple coneflower)

This has been shown to have powerful anti-viral and anti-bacterial potential, so can be used where pain is associated with infection. It helps indigestion discomfort and relieves ulcer pains in the digestive tract. It is used as a pain-killer and reliever of symptoms of haemorrhoids.

Passiflora (passion flower)

A useful herb for treating restlessness, anxiety and irritability and for calming painful spasms. It is widely used to treat insomnia.

Half a teaspoon of its tincture (liquid extract) before meals and at bedtime is a usual dosage recommendation.

Peppermint

Used as a tea or in extract form extensively for stomach cramps and digestive upsets.

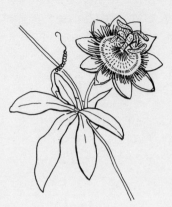

FIGURE 40 A passion flower.

Raspberry leaf

Used as a tea or in extract form for menstrual cramps.

Red sage

Used as a gargle (for sore throat, for example) adding a teaspoonful of fluid extract to a cup of water. Can also be used as a herbal tea.

Slippery elm bark powder

Be sure this is pure powder with no additives. This is ideal for soothing acute digestive disturbances. It is taken spoon by spoon as a gruel.

Viburnum opulus (cramp bark)

This is a well-known remedy for cramp and pain of a spasmodic nature (comes and goes) especially when these are the cause of irritability and mental distress. It is regarded as being more suitable for use in women.

Boil half an ounce of shredded bark in a pint of water and then leave to cool. A strained tablespoonful is taken before meals and at bedtime. Or half a teaspoonful of a fluid extract (from a herbal supplier) should be taken at the same times as for the infusion.

BACH FLOWER REMEDIES

The so-called 'Rescue Remedy' is suggested for use for its emotional calming effect after physical or emotional shock. Take a few drops in water every half an hour until an easing is noticed.

HOMOEOPATHIC REMEDIES

Homoeopathy, in simple terms, uses minute amounts of substances which, in larger doses, would give you symptoms very similar, or identical, to those you already have and want to be rid of. Because of their extreme dilution, homoeopathic remedies are very safe, carrying absolutely no danger of toxic reaction.

In true homoeopathic medicine the practitioner will find a remedy which fits not only your symptoms but your personality and constitutional make-up. However, in what is called 'emergency' or first-aid prescribing these constitutional factors are left out and only the symptoms looked at.

The following list is of the main remedies, some of which – such as Rhus tox – have recently received medical approval in stringent trials (Rhus tox was found effective in treating muscular pains and inflammations – something known to homoeopaths for over a century).

Cautions:
- If a homoeopathic medicine is taken for a symptom it should not be repeated unless the symptom continues unchanged or returns. If there is an improvement, allow this to continue of its own accord. In this instance it is a mistaken belief that because something helps, more of the same will help even more. In other words, homoeopathy's subtle remedies should be allowed to do their job.

- Avoid the use of strong-smelling substances (such as rubs and ointments etc.) when using homoeopathic remedies.
- It is important that homoeopathic remedies are stored in a cool dark place away from any fumes or aromatic smells which could damage their sensitive structure.
- The remedies should be taken between meals and allowed to dissolve under the tongue.

Note: The letters and numbers following the remedy name indicate the degree of dilution used, and it is important that you use not just the correct remedy but the correct 'potency' as indicated. Most Health Food Stores and many pharmacies now stock homoeopathic remedies in these potencies.

Aconitum 12X

For severe pains (e.g. following burns) one pilule.

Apis 12X

For insect bites and stings. One pilule every 30 minutes until pain/swelling eases.

Arnica 6X

Following accidents or injury. Take a pilule under the tongue every half hour until ease is noticed.

Arnica 3X

Following bruising take one or two pilules under the tongue every half hour.

Chamomilla 3X

For general anxiety and non-specific pain relief. Dissolve under the tongue whenever needed.

Hypericum 6X

For cuts and open wounds take one pilule every hour for three to four hours.

Rhus tox 6X

Take every hour when muscular pains (e.g. fibrositis) are strong.

CHAPTER TEN

Healing, Therapeutic Touch and placebo power

The laying on of hands, faith healing, spiritual healing and Therapeutic Touch, all have a common thread and all have shown, under clinically controlled conditions, that they can reduce pain and anxiety to a significant degree.

When such healing is applied, the person providing the treatment holds their hands in an area which they feel appropriate to the patient's needs, but their hands do not actually touch the patient – they are held some inches away from the surface. The healer then focuses attention on thoughts which are healing, soothing, supportive and compassionate, holding those thoughts for a matter of minutes before usually moving the hands to another position.

Just what happens is unclear, but in one fascinating Canadian study patients received exactly this method of treatment from nurses for the relief of chronic headache. A definite reduction of intensity of pain was recorded by these patients, and they were also shown to use far less pain-killing medication in the hours after treatment. This could well be put down to the placebo effect were it not for the fact that in this study an equal number of headache patients (a control group) received apparently the same treatment but in this case the nurses were doing mental arithmetic instead of thinking healing thoughts whilst 'laying on hands'. There was no reduction in pain or use of pain-killers amongst this group. Clearly, what the healer thinks makes the difference.

At McGill University in Canada research was conducted using dishes of enzymes or bacteria which had been damaged by exposure to radiation. When healing was applied, the damaged enzymes or bacteria were found to recover full vigorous activity, whilst those untreated continued to show poor activity. So, something which is not easy to explain can happen when healing thoughts are directed.

While it might be assumed that a prerequisite is that the patient receiving healing should *believe* that something positive is going to happen (should have faith, in other words), it has been found that this is not the case. Benefits have been recorded in sceptics as well as believers, and it seems that, whilst a belief in the treatment is always of help, what matters most in healing is what the healer is thinking at the time treatment is given.

THERAPEUTIC TOUCH

Many nurses in North America, and increasingly in the UK, have learned a form of healing technique called Therapeutic Touch for use in hospitals and general practices. The title is confusing since the patient is not actually physically touched.

PLACEBO POWER

As intimated above, if you believe something will relieve pain it is likely to do so far more readily and effectively than if you do not believe it can help. In double-blind trials involving over a thousand people suffering from chronic pain, relief was felt not just by those given pain-killing drugs but also by half of those in a similar size control group who thought they were being given such drugs but who were in fact receiving dummy pills (placebos).

In order to see just how impressive this is, consider that a 50 per cent reduction in pain levels was achieved by people taking placebo compared with people taking aspirin; and when compared with the relief obtained from morphine, the most powerful narcotic drug, the relief was still found to be around half the level of reduced pain. How could this happen? Because of the *anticipated* result, it is thought.

Drs Melzack and Wall explain: 'This shows clearly that the psychological context – particularly the physician's and patient's expectations – contains powerful therapeutic value in its own right in addition to the effect of the drug itself.'

In another research study it was shown that people who had previously shown themselves to be helped by placebo were relieved of nearly 95 per cent of their pain by morphine, while those who were not influenced by placebo only had around 50 per cent benefit from morphine. This shows us that whenever you take a pain-killer, around half of its benefit may be from the placebo effect alone, and that you would probably receive at least 50 per cent relief from pain by taking a dummy substance with no active ingredients if you were a placebo reactor.

Placebo facts

- Placebos are far more effective against severe pain than mild pain.
- Placebos are more effective in people who are severely anxious and stressed than in people who are not, and clearly their anti-anxiety effect is at least part of the reason for their usefulness.
- Placebos work best against headache-type pain (over 50 per cent effectiveness).
- In about a third of all people most pains are relieved by placebo.
- A placebo works better if injected than if taken by mouth.
- Placebos work more powerfully when they are accompanied by the suggestion that they are indeed powerful and that they will rapidly produce results.
- Placebos which are in capsule/tablet form work better if two are taken rather than one.
- Large capsules work as placebos more effectively than small ones.
- Red placebos are most effective of all in helping pain problems.
- Green placebos help anxiety best.
- Blue placebos are the most sedative and calming.
- Yellow placebos are best for depression, and pink are the most stimulating.
- Placebos have been shown to be effective in a wide variety of conditions, including anorexia, depression, skin diseases, diarrhoea, palpitations and many more.

- Placebo effects occur in other ways than by taking something by mouth or injection – for example, any form of treatment from manipulation to acupuncture to surgery carries with it a degree of placebo effect.

This in no way reduces the value of the treatment method being used, any more than we can say that because some of the pain-killing effect of morphine derives from the placebo effect that it is of no value as a pain-killing drug. Recognition of the placebo effect simply allows us to realize the importance of the power of suggestion on all of us – some of us being more influenced than others.

It is essential that we should not think that because a placebo fails to work for some people that they are not genuinely suffering pain, or that relief is falsely claimed by those for whom it works. We should see it as proof of the self-healing abilities of the body/mind which the dummy medication has released, and that our attitudes and emotions are powerful aids (or hindrances) to our own recovery. The bringing together of the feelings of hope and expectation with a relationship with caring helpers, professional or otherwise, can only assist in recovery or coping.

What we need to learn is the amazing power of suggestion, the direct and huge influence which the mind has over the nervous system and body as a whole. Part of the placebo benefit comes from the reduction in anxiety which is brought about by the knowledge that something is being done to deal with the problem. We can recognize the need therefore to try to achieve similar stress and anxiety reduction by use of appropriate tactics.

PART THREE

Options for specific conditions

This section gives specific advice on the following conditions, and offers a choice of treatment options. Each listed condition has a 'menu' from which choices can be made. It is not suggested that more than one self-help approach be tried at the same time. For example, if you were to treat a headache by dealing with trigger points, using hot and cold applications, taking herbal medicine and practising visualization all at the same time, it would be demanding and stressful, and consequently counter-productive. Use one method at a time and give it time to be effective before trying something else.

The order in which the conditions are listed is from head to toe.

Headaches, general
Headaches, migraine
Headaches, cluster
Sinus inflammation
TMJ (jaw) problems
Earache
Eye pain
Mouth and tongue problems
Toothache and gum problems
Sore throat
Arm pain
Raynaud's Syndrome
Chest pain (other than
  heart disease)
Heart pain
Back pain

Muscle and tendon problems
Joint pain
Nerve pain
Abdominal and digestive pain
Bladder and kidney pain
Gynaecological (pelvic) and
  menstrual pain
Childbirth
Varicose veins
Skin diseases
Abscesses and boils
Chilblains and frostbite
Cramp
Stings and bites
Burns and scalds
General/whole body pain

The following symbols have been used to indicate which treatments are suitable for self-application, and which are not:

S   Suitable for self-application
NS   Not suitable for self-application
ES   Best applied by an expert but can also be self-applied

When you apply any of the treatments listed as self-help you will need to refer to the appropriate chapter (such as Hydrotherapy, for example) for a full description of the method.

If the pain seems to be aggravated by the self-help treatment, stop using it and get expert advice. You may have used the method wrongly or inappropriately.

Never try to self-apply any of the treatments marked as requiring expert application. Always consult a suitably qualified practitioner.

In the recommendations for particular conditions, names of herbal or homoeopathic or other substances may appear which are not listed in the general text of the book. For example, Ignatia 3X is given as a homoeopathic remedy for tension headaches (when these are related to emotion). Although Ignatia is not in the general list of homoeopathic remedies in this book, its appearance here is not in error, but indicates that this particular remedy has a very specific use in this aspect of the condition but not a wider application.

HEADACHES (GENERAL)

Headaches can be roughly divided into:

1. Headaches with serious underlying causes
2. General headaches with uncertain causes
3. Tension headaches
4. Migraine headaches
5. Cluster headaches

1. Headaches with possibly serious underlying causes

See a medical practitioner as soon as possible if:

- your headache is accompanied by blurred vision, and the pain behind your eyes is strong
- you have headaches which are associated with a temperature
- your headache is accompanied by a stiff neck and you feel sensitive to light
- your headache came on after a blow or fall
- your headache comes on after taking prescribed medication
- your headache is accompanied by any of the following:
  persistent throbbing;
  worse for lying down;
  improved by being upright;
  partial loss of vision and/or accompanied by temperature
- your headache (forehead or temple area) starts following a sudden turning of the head.

2. Headaches with uncertain causes

Many headaches have 'general' causes or are accompanied by other symptoms – for example, constipation; overeating (especially of fatty foods); straining at stool; being at high altitude; problems associated with eyes, ears or teeth.

Use treatment and self-help methods as for tension headaches (see below) and eliminate causes.

Homoeopathic first-aid for general headaches-;

S   From overeating, combined with feeling of abdominal fullness: Pulsatilla 6X taken every hour until headache eases.-;

S   If headache follows a fall take Arnica 6X hourly and see a doctor.

S   If headaches follow sunbathing or heat exposure take Belladonna 6X until pain eases. This remedy is most useful if the headache is accompanied by a flushed face and throbbing head.

S   If the headache follows sun-exposure and is worse lying down, with pain at the back of your head/neck take Glenoine 6X hourly until relief is obtained. Meanwhile, see a doctor.

S   If there is indigestion and/or constipation along with the headache Nux vomica 6X taken night and morning for a few days should help.

S   If the headache is accompanied by fear or excitement related to anticipation, Gelsemium 6X taken hourly will help.

3. Tension headaches

Tension headaches start gradually and last for varied amounts of time, although they can be constant. It is not a pulsating pain, but usually dull with a sensation of pressure or tightness, either on both sides (temple area or forehead) of the head or at the back of the head.

Orthodox medicine

S   Over the counter pain-killing medication can be helpful in masking the symptom, but this does nothing to address the cause and can result in new problems such as stomach bleeding (if aspirin is used). All have potential side-effects, so use with caution.

Self-help first-aid

S   Often helped by adopting a position which eases the pain (sitting with head in hands, for example).

S   Tension headaches are aggravated by being cold/shivering, so keep warm.

Counter-irritant
NS Acupuncture

S TENS (pads sited on temples, or on either side of base of skull, or at base of neck, or in any position which masks the pain).

Healing/Therapeutic Touch
NS Can be very helpful.

Herbal
S Any of the herbs which are calming and soothing are useful, including chamomile and passiflora (as tea or herbal extract/tablet).

S Massage of the temple area with peppermint oil or menthol.

S Drink a tea made from ginger, chamomile, lavender or rosemary.

Aromatherapy
S Some essential oils can help headaches, especially if used early on. Chamomile and lavender both induce relaxation. Three or four drops of either of these (or a combination using two drops of each) added to a bath in which you soak for 30 minutes will reduce tension and may help your head.

Homoeopathy
S If there is a traumatic background (injury) Arnica 6X should be taken hourly until improvement starts.

S If headache relates to emotion Ignatia 3X is suggested hourly or until improvement starts.

Hydrotherapy
S The deep relaxation available from wet-sheet pack or neutral bath will help reduce tension headache pain.

S Hot and cold compresses to back of neck or . . .

S . . . cold compress to forehead or back of neck or . . .

S . . . hot application to back of neck/shoulders, followed by massage.

S Simultaneous hot foot bath can be used with any of the above.

Nutrition
S Light food or liquids only; especially if nausea is also present.

Manipulation and massage

ES Massage to neck/shoulders plus stretching of the muscles in this region by slow self-exercise or treatment.

ES Trigger point treatment if active triggers can be found. Most likely sites are in main neck muscles.

ES Acupressure points for headaches are found at base of skull and on temple just behind bone at side of corner of eye. Firm sustained thumb or finger pressure on these points for up to a minute at a time often eases head pain.

NS Osteopathic, chiropractic or physiotherapy attention may be needed for chronic problems.

Stress reduction

S Biofeedback and/or relaxation techniques for chronic headache problems have been shown to give individual ability to stop headache developing after about four weeks of training.

S Visualization is appropriate especially if Autogenic Training has been practised.

HEADACHE (MIGRAINE)

Migraine headaches usually start slowly, sometimes beginning with an aura of symptoms such as flashing lights in the 'classic' form, but there is often no more than a sense of nausea before the headache starts. The pain may last hours or days, is always one-sided in true migraine (usually around the temple/forehead/eyes) and may occur at intervals of anything from every few days to a few times a year. The pain is sharp, throbbing/pounding and severe.

The cause of migraine remains unclear, but the problem includes changes in circulation in the head, including dilation (expansion) of some blood vessels, local inflammation involving nervous system structures, and changes in the 'stickiness' of blood, making it more easy to clot. There are also psychological aspects to the condition in many cases. Migraines are more common in women, and it seems to be an inherited tendency.

Nutritional (see below) and other causes should be avoided where possible. Common predisposing factors include flickering or bright lights, or TV, weather conditions, stress (frequently following rather than during) and hormonal imbalances, especially around period time.

Orthodox medicine

NS A variety of drugs are used to control migraine. Some prescription medicines, such as ergotamine, give excellent symptom relief in some people, but not others. All drugs, prescription or over the counter, have side-effects and some have been shown to *increase* the likelihood of more headaches.

Use prescription drugs with caution at the beginning of a migraine or cluster headache, and if despite their use headaches seem more frequent or you seem to be needing more of them to relieve pain you might be reacting to the medication itself. Get expert advice from a pain or migraine clinic, but in general do not take ergotamine-based drugs more often than once in four days.

Self-help first-aid

S Holding (or lying on) something cold against the painful part of your head or base of your skull/neck area for 20 to 30 minutes gives many people instant relief.

S Lie down in a cool/dark room and apply *visualization/Autogenic Training* methods (warm hand/cool forehead).

S Pressure techniques (see below).

Counter-irritant

NS Acupuncture has a very good success rate in reducing frequency and intensity of migraines – not during an attack, though.

TENS has *not* had good results with this type of headache.

Healing/Therapeutic Touch

NS This can be extremely soothing during attacks, and can help prevent them.

Herbal

S Feverfew is a member of the chrysanthemum family and is remarkably effective in preventing migraine headaches. It is of no value during an attack. Tablets or capsules are available at pharmacies or Health

Food stores. To ensure that you get the active part of the plant, though, it is best to grow it (a window-box will do) and to chew one leaf daily (in a sandwich perhaps as the leaf is extremely bitter).

Aromatherapy

S   Some essential oils can help headaches, especially if used early on. Chamomile and lavender both induce relaxation. Three or four drops of either of these (or a combination using two drops of each) added to a bath in which you soak for 30 minutes will reduce tension and may help your head.

Homoeopathy

S   Iris 6X is a well-known remedy which can relieve the symptoms of migraine.

S   In children, sick headaches (which may be migrainous) are frequently relieved by use of Arsenic 3X, especially if the headache is associated with excitement, restlessness and/or vomiting.

Hydrotherapy

S   Ice pack to base of skull/upper neck can help abort an attack, but it will not help much once the migraine is fully active.

Nutrition

S   Possible causes of migraine which should be avoided until proved 'safe' include:

Alcohol.

Tyramine-rich foods. Mature cheeses, pickled herring, chicken liver, the pods of broad beans, tinned figs, chocolate and some nuts are all rich in this amino acid.

Nitrite-rich foods such as cured meats, hot dogs, bacon, ham, salami.

Low blood sugar (hypoglycaemia) which can result from missed meals or a diet rich in refined sugars and low in complex carbohydrates can trigger migraine. Regular (three or four) meals daily, plus snacks, which focus on adequate protein and complex carbohydrate (whole grains, fruit and vegetables) are suggested.

Other common foods which trigger migraine are those containing monosodium glutamate (MSG) which may be in Chinese restaurant food unless you specifically ask for it to be left out. Artificial sweeteners such as aspartame have been shown to produce more and more severe migraines in sensitive people. This is based on the amino acid phenylalanine and in large quantities (several sweetened drinks, for example) it has a chemical effect.

ES Specific nutrients have been shown to be deficient in some people with migraine, including magnesium. A trial of taking 500mg daily for a month will indicate whether this is helpful.

ES For women who have migraine attacks around period time, a supplement of vitamin B6 (100mg daily) and vitamin E (200mg daily) as well as the magnesium (400 to 500mg daily) often helps prevent this symptom of hormonal imbalance.

Manipulation and massage

NS Osteopathic and chiropractic treatment can relieve the frequency and intensity of migraines if the cause lies in spinal or other joint dysfunction. It is of little value during an attack, however.

ES Massage is useful to soothe associated tension in neck/shoulder muscles, and it assists in improved circulation/drainage.

ES Pressure on painful points can be useful. Key points:

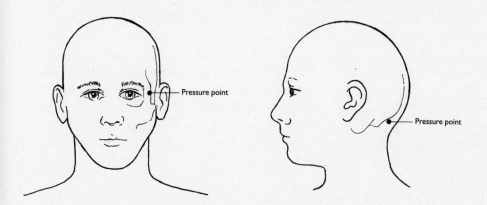

FIGURE 41 Two pressure points on the head: a) *left* just behind the bone between the temple and the eye, and b) *right* just below the rim of the skull.

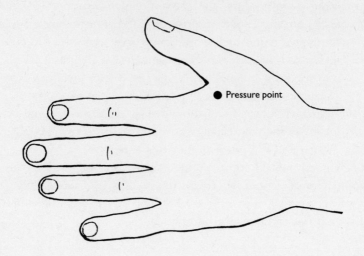

FIGURE 42 A pressure point between the index finger and thumb (it lies closer to the finger).

Two points which lie just behind the bone between the temple and the eye.

Two depressions at the top of the neck, just below the rim of the skull.

A point found between the index finger and thumb on each hand. Squeeze these together to find the highest part of the mound of muscle which this creates. Press into the muscle at this point, slightly towards the index finger. This should be tender. Trial and error will help you find these key points which relieve the head pain. Apply no more than mild pressure for seven to ten seconds at a time with short (three second) rest periods until the pain starts to abate. Do not continue for more than two minutes at a time or you could bruise the area.

Stress reduction

ES Biofeedback and relaxation exercises learned and practised between attacks can help reduce mechanical tensions which are associated with the headaches. They also allow application of deep relaxation when an attack is pending or in place, which can reduce severity.

ES Visualization and Autogenic Training are very useful. Again, these should be practised between attacks and used when they are coming on or present. The image of warm hands and/or cool head are the strongest mind messages for migraine.

Note: Biofeedback, Autogenic Training and use of TENS machines, while being ideal for self-application require that they be learned from a skilled teacher/instructor for optimum results.

HEADACHES (CLUSTER)

These, like migraine, are usually one-sided, but they differ in that they start very suddenly with no warning. It may last minutes or hours (usually about an hour) with a throbbing intense ('unbearable') pain focused in the eye, temple, neck and/or facial areas, perhaps going into the lower teeth and/or shoulder of the affected side. Cluster headaches are most likely to start in the early evening, between 6 pm and 8 pm. They tend to recur in frequent clusters and may be accompanied by flushing, sweating, running nose or tears. Men have them more commonly than women, usually first suffering them in their early 20s.

Research shows that the blood vessels in the eye become engorged/swollen, and that allergies may be involved in the cause.

Orthodox medicine
NS As in migraine, ergot-based drugs are commonly used. All drugs, prescription or over the counter, have side-effects, and some have been shown to increase the likelihood of more headaches.

Use prescription drugs with caution at the beginning of a cluster headache and if, despite their use, headaches seem more frequent or you seem to be needing more of the drug to relieve pain you might be reacting to the medication itself. Get expert advice from a pain clinic, but in general do not take ergotamine-based drugs more often than once in four days.

NS An alternative orthodox approach is the use of inhaled oxygen which has been shown to diminish intensity or to acutally switch off cluster attacks within a few minutes for a large proportion of patients.

Other drugs used include those which have an impact on the circulatory system. None are universally helpful and all have side-effects.

Self-help first-aid
In all respects as for migraine.

Hydrotherapy
S　Cold foot bath.
S　Hot foot and hand bath (using one teaspoonful dry mustard to two gallons of water if possible) together with cold/ice pack to neck/head.
S　Neutral bath at the very start of the headache.

SINUS INFLAMMATION

Orthodox medicine
Antibiotic treatment will be used in the acute phase if there is infection, and surgery to enhance drainage may be suggested in the chronic stages.

An allergic background is not uncommon in sinus problems, and this could be treated with antihistamine drugs – although these will actually dry the nasal passages and cause any mucus obstruction to become thicker and more difficult to drain away. The acute phase is very painful indeed, and pain-killing medication may also be prescribed.

Over-the-counter sinus 'cures' (sprays etc.) which alleviate internal pressure by constricting the blood vessels may give symptomatic relief, but they do nothing to remove the cause of the problem, and they further irritate the mucous membranes of the sinuses, and impair drainage. If over-used these sprays can, make matters much worse, damaging the mucous membrane permanently.

Self-help first-aid
S　A very light diet is indicated when sinus inflammation is acute – such as citrus fruit only for up to 48 hours. Alternatively other fruit and/or salad only (raw diet) can be tried. If the sinus problem is because of an infection or allergy this approach will rapidly reduce catarrhal congestion.

S   Steam inhalations are useful in unblocking the sinus obstruction in the nose. Make a 'tent' with a towel over a steaming kettle or saucepan and expose your face and breathing channels to this humid, hot air for up to 15 minutes at a time, several times daily. Various aromatic plants or their oils can usefully be added to the steaming water, e.g. thyme, eucalyptus, pine or cloves – or the combination Olbas oil.

S   Ensure that the room you are in is humid by steaming a kettle in it regularly, or by using a humidifier.

Counter-irritant
NS   Acupuncture is helpful in chronic conditions.

Herbal
S   Garlic. Three to six capsules daily.

S   *Echinacea augustifolium* (highly recommended for all infections).

S   Aromatherapy oil of pine (for inhalation) or hyssop (for inhalation – see under Herbal heading in section on coughs).

Hydrotherapy
Note: Do not use ice on your sinus area as it will aggravate the condition.

S   Cold (warming) compress over the affected area using a knitted cap or something similar to hold this in place. This can be applied when going to sleep. It must become warm within a minute or two or it could irritate the condition. To ensure this, make the cold damp material (cotton) one layer only and wring it well out so that it is damp and not wet. Cover well with woollen material and then insulate with the cap. Leave on for an hour or more if soothing. Repeat several times daily.

S   A salt spray is also useful, applied up the nose from an atomizer spray. A tablespoonful of salt to a pint of warm water is the right strength.

S   Inhalation of freshly made beetroot juice (from raw beetroot). This should be held in the nasal passages for as long as possible (a minute or so) before being allowed to either run out of the nose or down the back of the throat. If possible, do not swallow this. Albeit messy and a bit unpleasant, it is remarkably soothing and healing.

S Alternatively, inhaling salt water and allowing it to run down into the throat before spitting it out is also helpful. The salt solution should be as above and warm.

Nutrition
S Vitamin A is needed whenever mucous membrane inflammation exists, and up to 50,000 iu daily can be taken. (Not for pregnant women.)
S Vitamin C up to 5 grams daily in divided doses.
S The enzyme bromelaine (from the pineapple plant) taken in doses of 1,500mg or more daily has an anti-inflammatory effect and is perfectly safe.

Manipulation and massage
NS Massage to the face and neck by an expert, accompanied by manipulation of the facial bones and neck assists in helping drainage from the congested area.
NS Cranial manipulation (osteopathic) is helpful in chronic conditions.

TEMPERO-MANDIBULAR JOINT (TMJ) PROBLEMS

Orthodox medicine
This condition is defined as a syndrome (cluster of symptoms) including pain and tenderness (when lightly pressed) of the muscles involved in chewing; noisy creaks and grating sounds from the joint on opening and closing of the mouth; and restriction of range of mouth opening. The condition affects 15 people out of every 100. Sometimes the condition relates to the muscles of the jaw, and at others to internal derangement of the jaw joint itself.

NS Dental and medical approaches to this widespread problem are seldom successful unless they take into account general body influences, including posture and habitual patterns of use in work and sport, as well as stress coping factors. A wide range of methods, including the use of special braces in the mouth, surgery, manipulation techniques and psychological methods such as relaxation are used with mixed rates of success. TMJ problems are usually aggravated by movement of the joint, and the muscles and the joint itself are very sensitive to pressure.

S Pain-killers such as aspirin are of short-term and limited value and they have side-effects.

NS Injection of procaine into trigger points in the neck, shoulders or face (points which on pressure reproduce the pain of TMJ) is very effective if followed by manipulation to relax the muscles involved. A condition which sometimes is confused with TMJ problems is inflammation of the trigeminal nerve (Tic douloureux). This is different in its type of pain (intermittent stabbing/electric shock-like pain rather than TMJ's fluctuating aching and radiating pain. Trigeminal neuralgia does not hurt locally when pressed, whilst TMJ does. When the pain is burning and throbbing and there is also flushing of the face with tears and running nose, it is probably a condition called vascular facial pain. Medical advice should be sought to decide which is which.

Self-help first-aid

See Hydrotherapy and Manipulation and massage below.

Counter-irritation

NS Acupuncture is very effective in relieving the pain if it comes from muscle sources, especially if trigger points are involved.

S Acupressure onto trigger points can be helpful, especially if followed by ice massage.

ES TENS is very helpful in relieving TMJ pain. It does not deal with underlying postural or dental causes, but it induces relaxation locally.

Healing/Therapeutic Touch

NS Can be helpful in chronic conditions.

Herbal

S Feverfew (*Chrysanthemum parthenium*) as a tablet or one or two leaves eaten daily (in a sandwich perhaps, as the leaf is extremely bitter) helps many joint problems.

Homoeopathy

S   Rhus tox 6X can relieve pain of muscular/joint origin.

Hydrotherapy

S   Place a hot towel over the jaw/face to cover the area for 10–15 minutes. Immediately follow this by massaging the area with ice for 90 seconds. Repeat once an hour.

S   Neutral bath or wet sheet pack will have a general stress reducing/relaxing effect and are therefore useful adjuncts to specific treatment.

Nutrition

ES   Supplementation with calcium and the B-vitamins can be useful.

Manipulation and massage

S   Self-massage of the painful muscles (slow circular movements with the tips of the fingers) with pressure applied to any particularly sensitive areas (5 seconds pressure then rest, repeat up to ten times) can relieve local muscle spasm and help circulation.

S   Massage of the neck and shoulders is also helpful as some of these relate directly to jaw mechanics.

S   Sit at a table with an elbow on the table and hand cradling your jaw. Try to resist with the hand as you open your jaw. Hold this isometric contraction for five to seven seconds, and then slowly and firmly open your mouth as widely as you can to stretch the muscles. Repeat several times.

S   Make sure you keep your jaw relaxed as much as you can, avoiding clenched teeth and grinding of teeth.

NS   Correction of chronic postural habits which are a major cause of TMJ problems requires attention from an osteopath, chiropractor or physiotherapist skilled in this work.

NS   Cranial osteopathy is also extremely useful.

NS   Re-education of posture may require lessons from a teacher of Alexander Technique or a Feldenkrais practitioner.

Stress-reduction methods

S   Deep relaxation of the body/mind has a beneficial influence on pain of the TMJ, especially if it involves relaxation of the neck and shoulder muscles as well.

Vibration (percussion analgesia)

S   Rapid low level vibration has been found to provide a speedy, safe and effective method for easing pain. A hand-held vibrator (from any pharmacy) is quite suitable for this purpose and may require firm pressure contact of the vibrator for up to half an hour before relief is noticed. Vibration should continue for 45 minutes at least. Relief of even chronic pain can then last for many hours, and in some instances for days. A high frequency works best (100Hz) if applied near to or below the area of pain.

EARACHE

If pain is because of inflammation of the middle ear it is more difficult to deal with than when the external ear canal is inflamed. To tell which is which before a doctor is seen, gently pull on the lobe of your ear and move it in various directions. If the problem is in the outer canal this will make the pain worse. If it is an inner ear problem (*Otitis media*) then movement of the ear will not make the pain worse.

Orthodox medicine

NS   Standard medical attention usually involves antibiotics (if infection is involved) or antihistamines (if allergy is present) plus pain-killing medication. In chronic conditions in children surgery is commonly used to try to improve drainage. There are times when the antibiotic approach is appropriate, but in many instances it is not (in fact, a number of research studies show it to be of no value in the acute phase of otitis) commonly leading to further problems, especially involving yeast overgrowth (which might be an underlying cause anyway) or to activity from more resistant strains of bacteria. Antibiotics may be more useful if the problem is chronic (six months or more). The surgical approach to otitis has only a limited record of success. A high proportion fail and require repeat surgery within months. Repeated operations can lead to hearing loss because of scarring.

Self-help first-aid

S   In cases of infectious earache soothing heat can be delivered to the ear from an oven-heated salt- or sand-bag applied to the area for half-hour periods, with a rest phase of half-an-hour between applications. Two pounds of salt in a muslin bag should be applied (wrapped in cotton) so that the affected ear lies on it or it lies on the ear. A partially heated, wrapped (in a tea towel) hot-water bottle can also be useful for this purpose.

S   If the earache is because of atmospheric changes (in an aeroplane, for example), chew gum, swallow frequently, suck a sweet, or hold your nose closed while gently blowing through it to 'pop' the eustachian tubes. Do not do this strongly.

S   If the earache develops soon after swimming (within minutes) hold your head at an angle so that the affected ear is downward, and hold two stones close to your ear and bang the stones together sharply to make a high pitched sound. The sound waves will often bring about a rapid release of the retained water.

Counter-irritant

NS Acupuncture is useful for dealing with chronic problems rather than acute ones.

S   Acupressure applied to a point which lies between the thumb and first finger in the fleshy mound close to the finger when these two digits are held together. Deep and sustained (for a minute or so) pressure here will hurt, but should relieve the ear pain.

Healing/Therapeutic Touch

NS Helpful in chronic conditions.

Herbal

NS If prescribed by a suitably qualified practitioner the use of the herbs Goldenseal and Echinacea (not for pregnant women) is helpful in safely dealing (without side-effects) with infections associated with ear problems.

NS Antiseptic herbals such as licorice, garlic and myrrh can all be helpful under professional guidance.

S   Put a few drops of warm almond oil or castor oil into the ears, especially if the problem is in the outer ear or relates to waxy build-up.

Homoeopathy

Depending on symptoms different remedies are indicated:

ES If the face is red and flushed: Belladonna 3X.

ES If the earache is recurrent and follows exposure to a draught, or in the early stages: Ferrum phos. 3X or 6X or Aconite 3X.

ES If earache follows measles or whooping cough: Pulsatilla 3X.

ES If there is restlessness and irritability: Chamomilla 3X.

Hydrotherapy

S A hot footbath can be soothing.

S Alternating hot and cold applications to the area around the base of the skull and neck can help improve local drainage and circulation.

S For *Otitis media* or general earache, obtain powdered charcoal from a pharmacy. Place three teaspoonsful of this, and the same amount of flaxseed (linseed) which has been ground in a blender together into a saucepan with a cup of water. Bring to the boil while stirring, and allow to cool down a bit. The mixture becomes jelly-like. Spread this over a square of paper kitchen towel so that the paste is about a quarter of an inch thick. Cover with another paper towel so that no paste comes out of the edges. Place, while still warm, over the ear so that it is moulded to the side of the jaw, covers the ear and extends to the hairline above the ear. Cover with a plastic sheet which extends beyond the edge of the paper, and bandage into place, leaving it there for up to ten hours. The whole poultice can be held more securely still by having a knitted cap or balaclava placed over it.

Nutritional

ES The defence mechanisms are helped by use of vitamin A (or beta-carotene its precursor, in doses of 15mg daily) and vitamin C (2–3g daily) and the mineral zinc (25mg daily).

NS Fasting is indicated and helpful if acute infection accompanies the earache. Water only (three to four litres daily for two days) – ideally under the guidance of a naturopathic practitioner – will usually help. Take advice before doing this without supervision.

S Avoid all sugar-based foods as these lower immune function.

Manipulation and massage

NS Specific cranial techniques applied by an osteopath can help eustachian tube drainage.

ES Massage to neck and upper chest can assist in this.

EYE PAIN

Orthodox medicine (and some first-aid measures)

There are various types of eye pain, and in ALL cases professional advice should be sought if eye pain does not go away within a few hours. Orthodox treatment will be aimed at the various possible causes using medication or surgery as appropriate.

(a) If there is sharp pain in the eyes it can be because of superficial damage or *irritation to the cornea*. The pain is characterized by sharp, stabbing and burning sensations which come on rapidly and which are felt below the upper lid. The eye will be sensitive to light and will be watering. Rubbing should be avoided. Tears which develop will normally wash the irritant away. If this is not rapidly achieved naturally, try to wash it away using cool boiled water. If this doesn't work, cover the eye with a loose bandage and seek help.

After removal of a foreign body (grain of sand etc.) or if there is a scratch/abrasion or if irritation is because of chemicals, such as chlorine in swimming pool water, use a solution made up of one part of calendula tincture in 25 parts of pure water to bathe the eye (use an eye bath).

Aconite 6 can be taken homoeopathically. Or, if the surface of the eye has been scratched, a drop of castor oil should be dropped onto the eyeball and the eye closed and covered with cotton wool and lightly bandaged.

Other causes of pain can include damage to the cornea resulting from disease. In all cases of rapid-onset eye pain, professional advice should be sought.

(b) In cases caused by *deep inflammation* the sensation is of a dull, sometimes severe, throbbing pain which seems to be inside the eyeball itself. It may also be referred to surrounding areas of the head and face. The pain may be constant or variable, and intense enough to prevent sleep. Vision may be reduced. The cause lies in inflammation of internal eye structures (iritis, keratitis and acute glaucoma are examples). Pain of this sort must be professionally dealt with as soon as possible.

(c) *Excess illumination* can cause pain or, more commonly, discomfort as a result of fierce glare (such as occurs when ultraviolet light or bright sunlight on snow is the cause). In some cases the light is less to blame than the normal screening mechanisms being faulty because of age or disease.

(d) In cases of *infection (or allergy)* affecting the eyes, such as blepharitis, the eyes will be red, irritated and gritty. A cold compress (see Hydrotherapy below) can be helpful.

Self-help first-aid

All cases described can be helped short-term by first-aid (as described) but most require medical or specialist assistance, especially in categories (b) and (c) above.

Counter-irritant

NS Acupuncture is helpful for chronic eye pain.

S Acupressure can help the discomfort of eyestrain (reading in poor light etc.):

> Place fingers or thumbs just to the side of the ridge where the bone above the eye meets the nose. Press steadily, but not heavily, on these points for up to a minute at a time. Repeat every half hour if necessary.

> A point will be found on either side of the head in a depression midway between the outer edge of the eyebrow and the outer corner of the eye, just behind the bone felt in that area. Press with fingers and thumbs for up to a minute at a time every half hour.

Healing/Therapeutic Touch

NS As in all cases, these methods can assist in chronic conditions.

Herbal

S Diluted calendula tincture (one part in 25 parts of pure water) used to bathe the eye and to apply to cotton wool which is bandaged to the closed eye is soothing after injury/irritation.

S For eyestrain from excessive or poor light, or use of inadequate glasses (wrong prescription), an infusion (as for making tea: place two teaspoonsful of the herb into a cup and add boiling water, allow to stand ten minutes, and use when cool) of the herb Euphrasia (eyebright) should be used in an eyebath and/or applied by compresses soaked in the liquid for 20 minutes every hour until pain and sensitivity eases.

S For styes, bathe the eye every four hours in *Hamamelis virginiana* (witch hazel) solution (one part witch hazel to four parts cool boiled water).

Homoeopathy

ES Arnica 6X taken every four hours for the first 24 hours after injury to the eye is very helpful.

ES In addition, if there has been severe trauma to the eye area involving the eye itself and/or its surrounding bone or tissue the remedy Symphytum 6X should be taken every four hours after the arnica has been stopped (after 24 hours).

Hydrotherapy

Note: Some eye conditions feel better for warmth, and others for being cooled. Allow your own judgement to operate in deciding which is most appropriate at the time.

An *eye compress* is best made by placing cotton wool into the bowl of a long-handled wooded spoon, and wrapping it in place with gauze bandaging. This is dipped into the hot or cold liquid – plain water or an appropriate herbal infusion or tincture (see above under Herbal) – and then gently squeezed to remove excess liquid before being placed gently over the affected eye. Apply such compresses for 20 minutes every hour until relief or professional help arrives. Hot applications help most in problems relating to the surface areas, and cold applications reduce congestion and soothe and relieve pain of a deeper nature (see Note above).

Manipulation and massage

NS Cranial osteopathy is useful in dealing with pain caused by structural problems if these arise from injury or birth trauma.

MOUTH AND TONGUE PROBLEMS

Orthodox medicine

A wide variety of medications for oral use are available over the counter and on prescription. All too often these deal with the symptoms and not the cause.

Mouth (canker) sores can result from yeast, virus or other infections (candidiasis, *Lichen planus*, herpes) and medical attention often focuses on these organisms. Teeth problems relating to poor denture hygiene, smoking or chewing tobacco can result in cellular changes (leucoplakia, erythroplakia) which receive specific medical attention (see note on denture hygiene under the Toothache heading).

Conditions such as diabetes, nutritional deficiency, hormonal deficiencies, especially in menopausal women, can lead to alterations in the mouth and tongue, resulting in pain.

Specific attention is required to deal with the **causes** of any of these problems in order to normalize the condition.

Self-help first-aid

S For rapid relief, hold a moistened (Indian) tea bag over the canker sore. The tannin is an astringent and also kills any yeast which might be involved.

Counter-irritant

S As for dental pain (see pages 149–50).

Healing/Therapeutic Touch

NS If available this can help ease the discomfort and distress of mouth and tongue pain.

Herbal

S   Plantago mother tincture applied locally by dabbing with soaked cotton wool to sore places in mouth.

S   Mouthwash with solution containing red sage (infuse the leaves as a tea) or tincture of myrrh (diluted five to ten drops in half a tumbler of warm water) or Aloe vera juice (five drops in a tumbler of water).

Homoeopathy

S   Plantago 3X.

S   Kreosotum 3X.

Hydrotherapy

S   An ice chip placed onto a tender canker sore can be helpful, as can sucking an ice cube if the mouth or tongue feels hot and raw.

Nutrition

NS   If yeast problems are involved, attention to this is needed systemically, as well as to local infestation of the mouth area. Professional advice is needed to deal with such problems comprehensively.

S   Chewing high potency acidophilus tablets helps, as does rinsing the mouth (and retaining for as long as possible – minutes if you can) a solution containing high potency acidophilus (Natren brand recommended) dissolved in warm water.

ES   Redness, soreness (and possibly scaling) at the junction of lips and the mucous membrane of the mouth (known as cheilosis) is often caused by vitamin B2 deficiency. Supplement with one yeast-free source B-complex tablet daily (taken at a meal time) as well as an individual supplement of 25mg vitamin B2 at a separate mealtime daily until symptoms vanish.

ES   Cracking and soreness at the corners of the mouth (angular cheilosis) may result from poor denture fitting or hygiene, as well as deficiencies of iron, folic acid, vitamin B2, B6 and/or B12. Supplementation can be attempted, but advice from a suitable professional is preferable.

ES   Tongue soreness also results from deficiency. Specifically, vitamin B2 (tip will be red and sore); B3 (produces fissures on tongue), and B6 (tongue tip red and sore). If the tongue is sore and bleeding this can mean vitamin C deficiency.

ES Aphthous ulcers can be caused by deficiency of iron, B12, B6 or folic acid.

NS All of the mouth and tongue problems mentioned can be the result of allergies, with wheat/gluten being one of the commonest. This needs professional guidance to assist.

Stress reduction

S All forms of relaxation will reduce perceived pain levels.

TOOTHACHE AND GUM PROBLEMS

Orthodox medicine

Dental attention, which should be sought as soon as possible. Pain relief from aspirin or other pain-killers, as well as oral pain-killing mouthwashes, can be effective short-term strategies, although they all have toxic side-effects. Do not place such pain-killers against the gum to ease pain as they can damage tissue unless sold as a mouthwash.

Self-help first-aid

S Local application of any of these, several times daily:
  Clove oil (nerve sedative);
  Brandy;
  Peppermint extract;
  Cinnamon oil.

Any one of these can be applied directly to gum/tooth margin or into tooth cavity if appropriate by use of soaked cotton-wool. Or cloves can be gently chewed to release their soothing oils.

S For pain/swelling of wisdom teeth, wash mouth frequently with salt solution. Salt water mouthwash (half a teaspoonful of salt to a tumbler of warm water) removes bacterial presence and is soothing.

S Or solution of tincture of myrrh (five to ten drops in half a tumbler of warm water) can be used as a mouthwash for toothache.

Counter-irritant

ES TENS is very effective in relieving all dental and gum pains.

NS Acupuncture is very effective in helping reduce pain levels:

A sensitive point on either index finger on the thumb side of the finger where the nail commences, close to the nail bed.

Just below the ankle bone on either leg, on the outer surface.

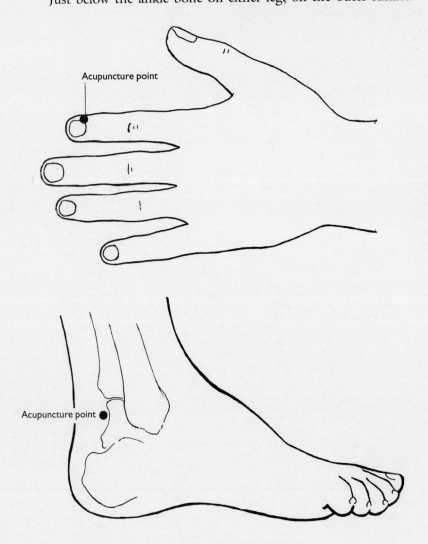

FIGURE 43 Acupuncture points for toothache and gum problems.

Healing/Therapeutic Touch
NS If available this can help ease pain and distress of tooth pain.

Herbal
ES Tincture of calendula diluted 50:50 with hot water and applied to painful, swollen gums (after dental surgery, for example) rapidly reduces swelling and pain.

Homoeopathy
S Chamomilla 3X or 6X (for neuralgia-like pains, especially if accompanied by restlessness and irritability). Ideal for children. The remedy can be taken half-hourly until relief is noted.
S Pulsatilla 6X (especially if accompanied by feeling weepy).
S Calcarea phosphorica 6X (if not helped by either of the above).
S Aconitum 3X (ideal if pain is burning/throbbing).

Hydrotherapy
S Massage outside of jaw with ice, on area overlying sore tooth, for rapid if short-term relief.
S Crushed ice in a plastic bag can be applied over painful tooth area (on face, not inside mouth) for ten to 15 minute periods every hour. Ideal for use after dental surgery or injury.

Denture hygiene
If dentures are causing pain have them seen to by an expert. They should be brushed daily with a denture toothpaste. At another time, after meals ideally, brush tongue with a gauze pad soaked in salt water and rinse mouth thoroughly with salt water. If plaque accumulates, soak dentures in a solution of one tablespoonful white vinegar to eight ounces of water. Fungal infections are common and can be helped by chewing high potency acidophilus tablets and using an antifungal solution for overnight soaking.

Stress reduction
S All forms of relaxation will reduce perceived pain levels.
S Breathing slowly and deeply is *always* helpful in reducing anxiety which makes pain seem worse.

Vibration (percussion analgesia)

S   Rapid low level vibration has been found to provide a speedy, safe and effective method for pain coming from inflamed dental structures. A hand-held vibrator (any pharmacy) is quite suitable for this purpose and may require firm pressure contact of the vibrator for up to half-an-hour before relief is strongly noticed. Vibration should continue for 45 minutes at least. Relief of even chronic pain can then last for many hours and in some instances for days. A high frequency works best (100Hz) if applied near to or below the area of pain.

SORE THROAT

Orthodox medicine

If it is because of infection, then antibiotics will almost certainly be used. Unfortunately, more infectious agents are becoming resistant to antibiotics, which also damage the delicate balance of friendly bacteria in our intestinal tract, creating other health problems. In children streptococcus micro-organisms are the commonest cause of sore throat of infectious origin (and sometimes in adults). Symptoms will be high temperature (over 102 deg F/39 deg C), swollen glands in the neck and white spots on the back of the throat and tonsils. In adults, various viruses (such as the common cold) and the yeast *Candida albicans* are common causes of sore throat. Most get better with or without treatment.

If sore throats are chronic, frequently recurrent and relate to tonsils, then surgery may be suggested. Removal of these should only be considered as a last resort. For example, if breathing is really difficult and there are many recurrences a year. Even then surgery is indicated only after trying conservative methods involving dietary exclusion (sugars, dairy products or other possible allergens) first.

Laryngitis, inflammation of the vocal cords is often because of dry, dusty or smoky atmosphere, or overuse of the voice. Preventive approaches (avoidance of causes mainly) are seldom difficult. Introduction of humidifiers in air-conditioned or centrally-heated homes is often all that is needed; or stopping smoking. In some instances throat pain can be serious, and if it persists or recurs frequently medical advice should be sought.

Self-help first-aid

S   Make sure you breathe through your nose, especially when outdoors, and if this is impossible cover your mouth with a scarf so that the air is filtered and warmer than would otherwise be the case. Ensure that the humidity of the room you are occupying is high (steam a kettle every now and then, or purchase a humidifier). There is nothing more irritating to an already sore throat than cold or dry air.

S   Gargles are a major help. See the suggestions under the Herbal heading, or use salt water to gargle regularly or irrigate and soothe your throat.

Herbal

S   Garlic taken in food or as capsules is powerfully antibiotic to yeasts, bacteria and many viruses. Take three to six capsules daily.

S   A teaspoonful of a solution of red sage extract (herbalist or homoeopathic pharmacy) in a cup of water is a marvellous gargle or mouthwash for sore throats and tonsillitis. Use several times daily. Or, for other forms of sore throat, gargle with any of the following:

    S   Geranium oil diluted three drops to a cup of warm water.
    S   Pine oil – two drops to a cup of warm water.
    S   Lemon juice – a small squeeze in warm water.
    S   Tea tree oil – three drops in a tumbler of water.

Homoeopathy

S   If the throat condition is part of the symptoms of a cold, then Nux vomica 3X (taken every hour until symptoms ease) is indicated (especially if it started after a chill and there is nasal discharge during the day but not at night, and there is restlessness and irritability and a feeling of not being able to get warm).

S   If the cold is worse in the evening and worse in a warm room, then take Allium cepa 3X half-hourly until symptoms subside.

S   If the cold is not triggered by a chill, then Arsenicum 3X taken half-hourly will usually abort it.

S   If accompanied by fever and tonsils are very red: Belladonna 3X.

NS For other forms of sore throat a professional homoeopath would need to advise on appropriate remedies.

Hydrotherapy

S   Irrigation of the back of the throat with very warm (not hot) salt water is useful. Obtain a syringe and fill with warm salt water. Lean over a basin and squirt this quite strongly onto the back of the throat, washing and irrigating the tender tissues. Use up to a pint of water this way, allowing the 'run-off' to exit the mouth (do not swallow it). Alternative constituents can include garlic oil (crush garlic into the water and strain through nylon stocking before use). This is ideal if the infection is a yeast such as Candida.

S   A cold (warming) compress applied to the throat overnight (as well as one around the abdomen if there is any temperature) helps soothe the soreness and drain the swollen lymph glands.

S   General body friction rub (skin brushing with a skin brush) helps detoxification and elimination functions. Useful in all infections.

Nutrition

S   A light (fruit only) diet or fast (water only) for 36 to 48 hours is the ideal treatment for all sore throats. Consult an expert if you plan on fasting for longer than that.

NS   If the infection is a yeast, then a specific low-sugar diet is required, combined with supplementation of 'friendly bacteria' such as acidophilus and bifidobacteria. Specialist advice is needed from a naturopath, a nutrition consultant or a doctor who uses nutritional methods of treatment.

S   Whatever infection is present, vitamin A (in the form of beta-carotene) in doses of 15mg twice daily, and vitamin C in doses of up to 5g daily (in divided doses through the day) are indicated.

Manipulation and massage

NS   Massage and manipulation of the neck and throat can speed resolution of throat problems. Consult an osteopath or massage therapist using lymphatic drainage techniques for this.

ARM PAIN

Thoracic outlet syndrome (TOS) or carpal tunnel syndrome (CTS)

The condition is one in which, usually through overuse or poor posture, pressure is brought to bear on the nerves which pass through a narrow channel in the wrist area (CTS) or running down from the neck under the collar bone (TOS). The pain of CTS is worse for use involving gripping and occupations with repetitive motions such as typing or writing. It is sometimes a numbness or tingling, sometimes accompanied by weakness in fingers and, when more severe, a burning ache. It may also be felt at elbow and shoulder. It is commonly eased by shaking the arm.

Orthodox medicine
Treatment will be by use of pain-killing drugs (sometimes cortisone injections), rest (splinting, for example) or physiotherapy, which may be helpful, or by surgery (to be avoided if at all possible) which is sometimes necessary to release the nerve if extremely tight fibromuscular bands are compressing the affected nerve.

Self-help first-aid
S   Rest from painful activities is essential, even if this involves splinting for a while.
S   Examine the way you work and alter it if at all possible. Take regular (hourly) breaks from routine to use hydrotherapy and gentle stretching exercises (see below) to relieve the tight structures.
S   Improve posture if you have TOS, perhaps by consulting a teacher of Alexander Technique for postural re-education.
S   Use ice massage on painful areas.

Counter-irritation
S   TENS is useful for either of these pains, but does not deal with the causes.
S   Acupuncture can relieve chronic pain and tension in muscles, but there must still be a new use of the arm/body or the problem will return.

Hydrotherapy

S   Ice massage over the entire arm is helpful.

S   Hot and cold applications (or bathing of) to entire arm, and specifically over lower neck/collar bone area (for TOS) and wrist (for CTS) helps circulation and muscle tone.

Nutrition

S   One of the easiest treatments for CTS is *sometimes* the taking of vitamin B6 since a deficiency of this vitamin brings on exactly these symptoms. Unfortunately, deficiency is not always the cause, but a trial for six to eight weeks should give the answer one way or the other. A dose of no more than 200mg daily should be taken with meals.

Manipulation and massage

ES   Massage of tense and tight tissues, plus stretching of any that are particularly tight, is a major help.

NS   Trigger point treatment is ideal if points can be found which, when pressed, reproduce the pain of the condition. Treatment of these by acupuncture, acupressure, ice massage, ultrasound, procaine injection or stretching of the muscle are all effective methods of eliminating the troublesome problems. This needs to be done by an expert.

NS   Osteopathic and chiropractic treatment can usually improve mechanical causes of this problem.

RAYNAUD'S SYNDROME

Orthodox medicine

Constriction of the tiny blood vessels in the hands and/or feet produces a characteristic change in colour (white), an intense coldness and pain. It is more common in smokers. Medical treatment concentrates on drugs such as calcium channel blockers (side-effects are headache and swollen ankles in some people) or surgery in which the nerve supply to the tiny blood vessels is cut (only done in extreme cases). Some drugs make matters worse, eg beta blockers used in blood pressure treatment and ergotamine used in migraine treatment can trigger Raynaud's symptoms.

Self-help first-aid

S Prevention is best, so keep warm (gloves, socks etc.) and avoid exposure to the air if it is really cold.

S Stop smoking, or avoid smoky locations if you are not a smoker.

S Rapid arm movement exercise can force blood through the tiny capillaries. Stand with your arms at your side and swing them strongly round and round (like a windmill) forward and up, and back and down, and forward and up . . .as high as you can, and as fast as you can (60 to 80 swings a minute). This often relieves hand symptoms in a minute or two.

Counter-irritation

NS Acupuncture helps chronic problems of this sort, but is of little use in acute stages.

Healing/Therapeutic Touch

NS Useful in chronic stages to improve tension states and circulation.

Hydrotherapy

S A method by which you can 'condition' your circulatory system is recommended by some experts, and has had success in large trials. Place two bowls with warm water in different environments – one in a warm room and one in a cold room, or outside in the cool. Dress as for indoors (lightly) and immerse your hands in the warm water indoors for between two and four minutes. Go to the outside (or 'cold' room) and do the same, but this time for eight to ten minutes. Go to the 'warm' room and repeat the first immersion. This triple immersion (warm room, cold room, warm room) should be done not less than four (ideally six) times a day, every other day until the symptoms of Raynaud's syndrome abate markedly. The conditioning process involves your body getting used to having warm hands in a cool atmosphere.

Nutrition

S Avoid coffee, as this constricts blood vessels.

S Try taking EPA (eicosapentenoic acid) capsules (three to six daily) for at least three months, as these can reduce the tendency for blood to become 'sticky'. In trials of the efficacy of EPA, half the people studied displayed better circulatory access to the extremities.

S   The following supplements are useful for anyone with circulatory problems:

nicotinic acid (vitamin B3) – 50mg three times a day after meals;
vitamin C – 1g daily;
vitamin E – 600 iu daily;
EPA as above, plus 1,000mg of evening primrose oil;
magnesium – 400mg daily.

Manipulation and massage

NS Osteopaths and chiropractors claim success in treating this condition by working on the neck and upper spinal structures to improve nerve and circulation supply.

NS Massage on a regular basis can assist in normalizing circulatory flow and relaxing tense structures in the neck and shoulder area.

Stress reduction

NS One of the most useful measures for anyone with Raynaud's syndrome is application of biofeedback methods which focus on circulatory markers (temperature of the hands etc.).

NS Autogenic Training focuses on warmth of hands and feet as part of its methodology and is very useful in helping to develop control over these states.

CHEST PAIN (OTHER THAN HEART DISEASE)

A study of hundreds of people taken to emergency rooms with what appeared to be a heart attack showed that around half of them had perfectly normal hearts and arteries. They were suffering from pain because of intercostal spasm (the small muscles between the ribs) brought on by poor stress response in that they were using their breathing 'machinery', notably the muscles, excessively and incorrectly, usually involving hyperventilation.

Test yourself to see whether you might have such a tendency. Sit comfortably, leaning back in the chair, and rest one hand on your abdomen above your umbilicus, and the other on your upper chest. Take a slow deep breath and note whether your chest hand or your abdomen hand is moving first, and which is moving most. If it is the chest hand, then you have a tendency to breathe in a way which could lead to chest pain when you are under stress. Pain may be localized in the muscles which hurt, or may be referred to the chest from trigger points in muscles in the back, abdomen or neck.

Self-help first-aid
S Slow deep breathing, involving the diaphragm, is essential. The timing is also important. You should inhale fully (into the lower chest so that your abdomen bulges slightly as you breathe in) to a slow count of two. You should then exhale slowly to a count of four or five. Repeat this many times until it becomes normal, and without strain. (See 'Anti-Arousal Breathing Technique', page 50.)

Counter-irritation
NS Acupuncture is very effective in helping restore breathing function by relaxing the tight muscles and dealing with any trigger points associated with the pain.
ES TENS can help relieve chronic chest pain.

Herbal
S Irish moss if there is a hard and bronchial cough.
S Hyssop aromatherapy oil (two drops to a basin of hot water) for ten minute inhalation (drape a towel over your head to contain the steam).

Homoeopathy
To treat an associated painful cough:

S If almost gagging when coughing: Ipecacuanha 3X.
S If cough is dry and violent: Nux vomica 3X.
S If cough is painfully hard: Pulsatilla 3X.

Hydrotherapy
S Cold (warming) compresses help to relieve intercostal spasm and tightness.
S Full sheet pack.

S　Neutral bath.

S　Local ice massage over painful areas or over trigger points which are sending pain messages to the chest.

Manipulation and massage

NS　Osteopathic and chiropractic attention to the spine, ribs and associated muscles is essential to normalizing problems caused by long-term overuse through poor breathing and postural habits.

NS　Massage of the muscles associated with breathing and the intercostal muscles assists in normalizing these, especially if trigger point activity is contributing to the problem.

NS　Soft tissue stretching using Muscle Energy Techniques helps normalize tight short muscles.

NS　Acupressure massage to trigger points or local tight areas is useful.

Stress reduction

NS　Biofeedback methods are helpful in restoring control over habits which have become well established.

NS　Hypnosis can help restore a less tense use of the 'machinery' of breathing.

S　Deep relaxation following on from breathing exercises (such as mentioned above) helps remove the underlying cause of the problem.

ES　Yoga stretching exercises can help restore normal function.

HEART PAIN

Orthodox medicine

If pain in the chest is because of a heart attack, crisis medical care will offer treatment which will include oxygen, nitroglycerine tablets, patches which relieve the immediate spasm, and an array of drugs which open up the circulatory channels tó the heart.

CAUTION: If you develop pain in the chest associated with being out of breath, sweating and nausea, and with pain radiating up into your throat/jaw (or centre of your back) or in the centre of or across your chest and into or down either arm, seek emergency medical attention immediately. It may not be a heart attack, but if it is, the sooner professional help reaches you the better.

But is it a heart attack?

Angina pain stays the same when you take a deep breath, so if yours gets worse, or better, on deep inhalation the chances are that what you have is caused by muscular or joint problems in the chest rather than by your heart. If the chest pain you have is worse for deep breathing it could be pneumonia, but is more likely to be a muscle/joint/spine problem.

If any pain in your chest worsens when you are resting, it could be caused by indigestion or inflammation of the pericardium around the heart, and a medical diagnosis is called for. Heart problems are not suitable conditions for self-treatment in the acute phases, although nutritional approaches and exercise are often remarkably effective in restoring heart function in the chronic stages, but they do require expert guidance.

Alternative care

NS Arterial disease which leads to many heart problems is often improved by use of chelation therapy. This uses an artificial amino acid infusion (called EDTA) into the veins to slowly unblock arterial narrowing. This safe method is available under medical direction in most countries despite still not being accepted by mainstream medicine.

ES It is usually applied in conjunction with dietary and exercise programmes, breathing retraining and stress reduction methods. Unlike medical approaches which use calcium channel blocking drugs to ease heart stress, alternative approaches lay emphasis on the use of magnesium, supplemented or injected, which is a natural calcium antagonist. Medical research has recently supported this approach, and it is cheaper and safer than the use of drugs. Additional heart help is available from a range of herbs, including garlic which offers remarkable benefits both in prevention and treatment.

BACK PAIN

Orthodox medicine

Bed rest, pain-killing and muscle relaxing medication, and possibly physiotherapy, traction or even surgery. These are the standard approaches. There is an increasing recognition by orthodox medicine of the value of conservative manipulation methods (chiropractic and osteopathic), and a number of research studies have found them to result in faster improvement than standard care.

If the pain (or numbness and tingling) extends down your leg to your foot, get professional advice, as you may have a herniated disc pressing on a nerve. If your back problem is associated with loss of bladder or bowel control, seek professional advice. If you are using self-help methods and improvement is not apparent within a few days, seek advice.

Self-help first-aid

S   Lie down on a firm surface if the problem is acute, either on your back or your side, but always with bent knees.

S   If you can lie on your back, bend your knees and slowly try to bring them (one hand on each knee) towards your shoulders. This stretches the muscles in spasm. If this hurts, stop at a point just before the pain, and let the muscles get used to the position.

S   Use an ice spray, or ice itself, on the painful area for five minutes every half hour. After each application, get back to the stretch position . . . as long as it is painless. Stay in that position for as much of the time that you can. Sometimes this is easier to do lying on your side (pillow between the knees).

S   Alternating hot and cold. A hot towel over the area renewed several times over a 20-minute period, followed by cold application, can 'break' a spasm.

S   Take a pain-killing medication if you cannot achieve comfort, and try to rest until the very acute phase is over.

S   Apply local pressure to sore spots within the area of pain. If you cannot reach these easily, place a tennis ball on the surface on which you are lying and get this to press for you. If it is painful alongside the spine, put two tennis balls into a sock and tie it. Lie so that your spine is between the balls, and gently move around to 'massage' the painful area.

Counter-irritant

NS   Acupuncture achieves very good results with acute and chronic back pain.

NS   TENS is very effective in relieving chronic back pain, although this may only be temporary if the underlying 'mechanics' are not sorted out.

Healing/Therapeutic Touch

NS These methods have provided remarkable degrees of relief in chronic back problems.

Herbal

S Bromelaine (pineapple plant extract) is a powerful enzyme which reduces inflammation safely. Take 2–3g daily during the acute phase of back problems, and half that amount during the chronic phase.

S Aromatherapy oils are useful, either massaged into the area, or in baths. In particular: chamomile, cypress, eucalyptus or rosemary – three to four drops of any of these added to a bath, or to an eggcupful of almond oil (for massage) is suggested.

Homoeopathy

S Rhus tox 3X every two hours until relief is achieved (especially if the pain is due to strain, but also if it is more of a muscular than a joint problem).

S Ruta 3X for bruised bones and tendons.

Hydrotherapy

See above under Self-help first-aid.

S Alternating hot and cold.

S Local ice massage.

S Cold (warming) compress overnight.

S Wet sheet pack for several hours during the day if you can lie straight.

S Hot Epsom salts bath in chronic back pain cases. 1 lb Epsom salts and ½lb common salt to a bath. Soak for 20 minutes and go straight to bed afterwards.

S Use of aromatherapy oils as indicated in Herbal above is suggested.

Nutrition

S Vitamin C in doses of 3–5g daily helps some people enormously when pain is acute. This should be continued indefinitely if disc problems are diagnosed, as it helps restore connective tissue structure.

S Calcium (1g daily) and magnesium (500mg daily) are suggested in chronic cases of backache, especially if there is associated spasm.

Manipulation and massage

NS Osteopathic or chiropractic care as soon as possible if acute.

NS Skilled therapeutic massage as soon as possible if acute, and frequently if chronic, using suitable oils (see Herbal above).

NS Soft tissue manipulation using Muscle Energy Techniques to stretch shortened structure if chronic, and Strain-Counterstrain methods if acute.

NS Acupressure (Shiatsu) for chronic problems.

Stress reduction

ES Biofeedback can help achieve relief of long-term muscular contraction.

ES Autogenic Training helps achieve deep relaxation, which in turn relieves back pain in many instances.

NS Hypnosis often achieves success in treating chronic back problems.

ES Yoga stretching methods for long term recovery.

NS Alexander Technique for postural re-education.

Vibration (percussion analgesia)

S Rapid low level vibration has been found to provide a speedy, safe and effective method for easing pain. A hand-held vibrator (any pharmacy) is quite suitable for this purpose, and may require firm pressure contact of the vibrator for up to half-an-hour before relief is strongly noticed. Vibration should continue for 45 minutes at least. Relief of even chronic pain can then last for many hours, and in some instances for days. A high frequency works best (100Hz) if applied near to or below the area of pain.

MUSCLE AND TENDON PROBLEMS

How do you know if it is a muscle or tendon problem? A strain occurs when a soft tissue is overstretched or overused, and a sprain occurs when the same thing happens very quickly (as when you turn an ankle).

When muscles are overused or abused they become stressed and quite often inflamed, as do the tendons which anchor them to bone. Injury such as a fall, wrench, twist etc. can be the cause, as can repetitive minor stress caused by overwork or postural misuse. One way to be sure that the problem is actually in the soft tissues and not the joint itself is as follows:

If movement hurts (as it almost always does with muscle or tendon problems), or if movement in a particular direction is restricted, carefully note which movements are the most uncomfortable. Say this is bending your arm, or raising the arm above your head forwards, or turning your head to one side, you should next see whether the same pain exists when that same movement is performed for you with you making no effort at all. For example, if turning your head hurts (or it is restricted) when you do it, sit relaxed and let someone else gently take your head in precisely the same direction. If it still hurts or is restricted, then the problem is in the joint not the soft tissues. If it no longer hurts, or is restricted when someone else moves it in the opposite direction, then it is indeed a soft tissue (muscle) problem.

Tendon problems will usually be aggravated when a static contraction exists. This means that if you cannot turn your head to the left without pain, trying to turn it while that movement was being resisted would be more painful if the cause was in the tendons.

Trigger points

Many pains in the muscles and joints of the body are referred to where they are felt by irritated local areas in muscle called trigger points. When these are pressed, the pain is felt at a distance, as well as locally in the trigger. If a pain exists which does not become aggravated when the area in which it is felt is pressed, then it may be coming from a distant trigger. Treatment of these by an expert (osteopath, acupuncturist, massage therapist etc.) can be through procaine injections, pressure techniques, acupuncture, ice massage or other methods, and usually needs stretching of the muscles as part of the treatment to normalize the condition.

Orthodox medicine

NS Pain-killers, anti-inflammatory medication, hydrocortisone-type injections and physical therapy. Only the latter methods address the causes, and are usually very successful if the actual problem in the soft tissues can be identified.

ES Immobilization by bandaging, and rest of the area, can speed healing in serious injuries.

Self-help first-aid

S   If you can walk on, or use, an area which has been injured, try self-treatment for two days, and if it is improving well just continue doing whatever is helping. If it is not a lot better within 48 hours, see a professional for advice and help.

S   If it hurts to use, rest it.

S   Ice massage (10–20 minutes every hour) followed by gentle stretching of the area.

S   Hot and cold alternating applications.

Counter-irritation

NS   Acupuncture is very useful in treating all muscular and tendon problems, especially if chronic. Ideal for trigger point pain.

ES   TENS is useful as a way of easing pain, acute or chronic, in soft tissues.

S   Acupressure is helpful. Seek tender/tight areas in muscles and apply pressure to these for 30 seconds at a time to see whether the whole area feels easier afterwards. Useful for treating trigger point pain.

Healing/Therapeutic Touch

NS   Helpful in chronic conditions, but can ease acute stages as well.

Herbal

NS   Herbs which can ease muscle spasm or irritable muscle conditions include:

> *Viscum album* (mistletoe)
> *Passiflora incarnata* (passion flower)
> *Scutullaria lateriflora* (skullcap)
> *Valeriana officianalis* (Valerian).

S   Aromatherapy oils are useful either massaged into the area or used in baths – in particular chamomile, cypress, eucalyptus and rosemary. Add 3–4 drops of any of these to a bath, or to an eggcupful of almond oil (for massage).

Homoeopathy

S   In case of recent injury Bach Rescue Remedy.

S   For bruised muscles: Arnica 3X in acute phase (first 24–36 hours).

S   If there is deep bruising or a muscle tear: Ledum 3X should be taken for a few days.

S   For all muscle aches and pains, as well as sprains affecting ligaments, especially when chronic: Rhus tox 3X.

S   For wrenched tendons or inflamed ligaments: Ruta 3X or as mother tincture rubbed into area.

S   If Ruta applied locally and taken internally in 3X potency fails to help tendon insertion pains, then Symphytum used the same way might (mother tuncture rubbed in and 3X potency taken every four hours).

Hydrotherapy

S   Hot and cold compresses after massage.

S   Ice massage before or after massage or as treatment of trigger points.

S   Cold (warming) compress left on overnight, followed by stretching or massage.

S   Before massage apply hot wet towel to area for five minutes.

S   Epsom salts bath or aromatherapy bath (see list of oils under Herbal above).

Nutrition

S   In all inflammatory problems a combination of EPA (fish oil) capusles (3–6 daily) and evening primrose oil capsules is helpful.

ES Food intolerance can be a cause of muscular pain. This needs to be eliminated (wheat is commonly a cause) and any deficiencies dealt with (vitamin B6 and magnesium deficiencies are common).

Manipulation and massage

NS Osteopathic soft tissue treatment should be obtained as soon as possible in all cases of muscle or tendon damage/injury unless they normalize within a few days.

S   Seek out tender areas in muscles opposite those which were stretched or strained, and while holding a pressure which hurts slightly, slowly and gently see if you can alter the position of the joint or area so that the pain goes out of the tender point being pressed. If you can find such a position, hold it for a minute or so, and retest the movement of the area; it could prove very much easier.

NS Osteopathic or massage treatment of trigger points.

S   Massage and self-massage to muscles to relax tissues and to encourage circulation, speeds normalization and eases pain. Use in combination with hydrotherapy.

Use of aromatherapy oils (see Herbal above) can be helpful.

S   After use of hot moist application stretching of muscle to pain-free limit is useful.

Stress-reduction

ES   Deep relaxation methods (Autogenic Training, for example) can help relieve chronic muscle problems, since emotional and physical stress both reflect on the soft tissues of the body.

Vibration (percussion analgesia)

S   Rapid low level vibration has been found to provide a speedy, safe and effective method for easing pain. A hand-held vibrator (any pharmacy) is quite suitable for this purpose and may require firm pressure contact of the vibrator for up to half-an-hour before relief is strongly noticed. Vibration should continue for 45 minutes at least. Relief of even chronic pain can then last for many hours, and in some instances for days. A high frequency works best (100Hz) if applied near to or below the area of pain.

JOINT PAIN (ARTHRITIC AND OTHER CAUSES)

Orthodox medicine

Pain around a joint may in fact be from muscle. How can you tell if it is a joint problem or a muscular problem affecting the joint? If, when you move the joint in a particular direction (say bending the knee), it hurts or is restricted, and if it also hurts or is restricted when someone else bends it for you . . . then it is a joint problem. As mentioned in the section on muscles, if something hurts or is restricted when you move it in one direction, and hurts or is restricted when someone else moves it in the *opposite* direction, then it is a muscle problem. If the problem in the joint is injury, then time and manual methods (physiotherapy, exercise and rest) usually corrects it. If it is arthritic, then a wide range of medications and surgical approaches are available. Some of these can be very helpful, while others (steroids, for example) can achieve major relief, but have the potential to do great harm.

Even the non-steroidal anti-inflammatory drugs (NSAIDs), commonly given for less serious joint pains and stiffness, are now known to actually have a long-term negative effect, over and above the digestive problems they commonly cause. In recent research, arthritic joints not treated at all over a 15-year period were compared with arthritic joints of people treated with standard NSAIDs, and the findings show that the untreated people retained much better use of their damaged joints with less pain and stiffness, and on x-ray there was far less damage to the joint surfaces. The lesson is that inflammation is part of the body's defence mechanism and it should not be damped down by drugs for anything but short periods or problems become more serious in the long term.

Trigger points
Many pains in the muscles and joints of the body are referred to where they are felt by irritated local areas in muscle called trigger points. When these are pressed, the pain is felt at a distance as well as locally in the trigger. If a pain exists which does not become aggravated when the area in which it is felt is pressed, then it may be coming from a distant trigger. Treatment of these by an expert (osteopath, acupuncturist, massage therapist etc.) can be through procaine injections, pressure techniques, acupuncture, ice massage or other methods, and usually there is need for stretching of the muscles, as part of the treatment, to normalize the condition.

Self-help first-aid
S   Ice massage or compress, followed by gentle pain-free movement.
S   Hot and cold alternating compresses if there is swelling, followed by gentle pain-free stretching.
S   Massage area with capsicum cream.

Counter-irritation
NS Acupuncture is extremely helpful in joint pain problems, especially if chronic, and for dealing with trigger points.
ES   TENS is a safe method of easing pain, acute or chronic, in joint problems.
S   Rubbing the skin over a painful joint with ointments containing various paprika (capsicum) extracts (to heat the area) is a helpful short-term measure.

Healing/Therapeutic Touch

NS Chronic problems in particular respond well to these healing methods.

Herbal

S Aromatherapy oils are useful, either massaged into the area or used in baths – chamomile, cypress, eucalyptus or rosemary. Add three to four drops of any of these to a bath, or to an eggcupful of almond oil for massage, for gout or arthritis.

S Herbs such as feverfew (gout and arthritis) and 'Devil's Claw' (*Harpagophytum procumbens*) taken regularly reduce arthritic pain levels substantially.

Hydrotherapy

See Self-help first-aid above.

S Ice massage, ice compress, hot and cold compresses in acute stages.

S Cold (warming) compress overnight in acute or chronic problems.

S Epsom salts bath or aromatherapy bath (see Herbal above).

Nutrition

S Taking EPA (eicosapentenoic acid) capsules has very beneficial effects on arthritic joint problems, and reduces inflammation safely.

S Evening primrose oil has an anti-inflammatory effect in joint problems such as rheumatoid arthritis, and can be taken along or in combination with EPA.

S Following a low animal fat/low meat/low sugar diet reduces inflammatory activity and pain in arthritic conditions.

S Fasting (under supervision if for more than 48 hours), on water only, helps reduce joint pain of rheumatic origin.

S Studies have shown that wearing copper bracelets has a significant effect in reducing arthritic pain. Some copper is absorbed through the skin.

S Cider vinegar and honey reduces arthritic activity.

NS If gout is the cause, a specialized diet is required.

NS In chronic and acute states of both rheumatoid arthritis and ankylosing spondylitis, improved status of the bowel achieved through fasting and a vegetarian diet, or an extremely low refined carbohydrate diet combined with high complex carbohydrate (vegetables, pulses) and adequate protein, have reduced pain and slowed progression of the diseases in well conducted medical studies.

Manipulation and massage

NS Osteopathic or chiropractic treatment is indicated in all chronic joint conditions, and as soon as possible after injury or strain in acute conditions.

NS Therapeutic massage helps to relax tight muscles, reduce congestion and improve circulation to joints in pain or restriction, and can be very useful.

NS Soft tissue manipulation and/or massage is indicated for trigger point relief if this is the cause of joint pain.

S Self-massage is also possible in many cases if the hands can reach the affected part. Use of aromatherapy oils (see Herbal above) is encouraged.

Stress reduction

ES Autogenic Training exercises and all forms of deep relaxation improve function of joints and reduce pain levels.

NS Hypnosis is helpful in many chronic joint conditions.

S Yoga stretching is extremely useful for stiff joints (as long as pain is avoided when doing exercises).

Vibration (percussion analgesia)

S Rapid low level vibration has been found to provide a speedy, safe and effective method for easing pain. A hand-held vibrator (any pharmacy) is quite suitable for this purpose, and may require firm pressure contact of the vibrator for up to half an hour before relief is strongly noticed. Vibration should continue for 45 minutes at least. Relief of even chronic pain can then last for many hours, and in some instances for days. A high frequency works best (100Hz) if applied near to or below the area of pain.

NERVE PAIN

Orthodox medicine

Nerve pain (which includes burning, tingling, pins-and-needles and other pain sensations) has a vast number of different causes, ranging from the pain in a limb which has been amputated (phantom limb pain – see Vibration heading below) to the host of neuralgic (irritation of a nerve) and neuritic (inflamed nerve) conditions. There are many and various causes of these, ranging from injury and infection (such as shingles) to malignant (cancerous) and arthritic changes. There are also many causes for the many different neuropathies resulting from diabetes, infection, nutritional deficiencies, alcohol toxicity, inherited factors and many other causes.

Another source of nerve pain is damage to part of the nerve root near the spine causing a distribution of pain and other symptoms (numbness etc.) along the course of the nerve. A typical example of this is compression of the sciatic nerve between discs in the low back. It is impossible in this book to classify the complex range of nerve problems which can cause pain. Treatments range from medication or local anaesthetics to surgery and, increasingly in pain clinics, to the use of acupuncture, TENS and counselling/stress reduction. Diagnosis by a neurologist is needed to sort out just what is happening in many cases.

Self-help first-aid

Note: Sometimes, but rarely, pains from nerve structures seem to get a little worse following some of the methods listed below. This does not necessarily mean you should discontinue the method, because experience is that improvement often follows. However, if in any doubt, get advice from an expert.

S   Neutral bath. This is the safest way of ensuring overall reduction in sensitivity of nerve structures and achieving mental calming at the same time. The bath water must be at body heat, and you can stay in it for hours if necessary (someone needs to do the topping up to keep the water temperature at blood heat, using a bath thermometer to check every few minutes).

Counter-irritant

NS Acupuncture for all nerve pains.

ES TENS is invaluable for relief of most, but not all, nerve pains. In some conditions, such as post-herpes neuralgia, there have been good and bad reports (bad meaning no benefit).

Vibration (percussion analgesia)

S Rapid low level vibration has been found to provide a speedy safe and effective method for easing phantom limb (and other) pain since the time of the American Civil War. A hand-held vibrator (any pharmacy) is quite suitable for this purpose and may require firm pressure contact of the vibrator for up to half-an-hour before relief is strongly noticed. Vibration should continue for 45 minutes at least. Relief of even chronic pain can then last for many hours, and in some instances for days. A high frequency works best (100Hz) if applied near to or below the area of pain.

Herbal

S Bromelaine (an enzyme extracted from the pineapple plant) in doses of up to 3g daily will reduce inflammation safely. It needs to be taken away from mealtimes throughout the day.

NS Herbal medication based on pulsatilla, Jamaica dogwood (especially for facial and sciatic neuralgia), passiflora, valerian, berberis, bryony, aconite and betony, may be prescribed by a trained herbalist or naturopath.

S Massage with Olbas oil, wintergreen, peppermint or myrrh.

S Chamomile as an essential oil can be used directly over the site of pain, in a bath (six drops in bath), or mixed with an eggcupful of almond oil as a carrier for massage.

Homoeopathy

S For neuralgia: Atropa belladonna (deadly nightshade) 6X.

S For nerve injuries: Hypericum 6X.

S If neuralgia brought on by cold: Aconite 6X.

Hydrotherapy

S Neutral bath as above.

S   Wet sheet pack.
S   Epsom salts bath.
S   Alternate hot and cold compresses.

Nutrition

S   Deficiencies of B-complex vitamins in general, and vitamin B12 in particular, commonly cause or aggravate nerve pain problems. A good quality supplement should be taken.

NS   Injection of vitamin B1 (100mg) and B12 (1mg) intramuscularly each week is suggested.

S   Calcium (1g daily in divided doses); magnesium (½g daily in divided doses; vitamin C in high doses(10g or more daily – to the level where diarrhoea starts) in divided doses, have all been shown to help where nerve irritation/inflammation exists.

S   Evening primrose oil (essential fatty acids): 1–2g daily.

S   A detoxification 'cleansing' diet of fruit only (apples and pears, for example) or vegetable juice (carrot/beetroot) for 48 hours is extremely helpful in many chronic nerve pain conditions, especially if there is a toxic or allergic condition aggravating it.

Manipulation and massage

NS   Cranial osteopathic attention is valuable for all neuralgic pain, such as Tic douloureux and Bell's palsy (a facial muscle paralysis).

NS   Skilled massage is helpful in many of the neuralgias, but needs to be extremely carefully applied.

Stress reduction

NS   Hypnosis can be useful to ease the perception of pain.

ES   Biofeedback, and stress-reducing methods such as Autogenic Training, can help reduce pain levels and provide you with an element of 'control' which lowers arousal and, in that way, allows greater tolerance of pain.

S   Breathing exercises (yoga pattern of two-second inhalation, five- or six-second exhalation) also lower arousal, reduce anxiety and allow greater tolerance of pain.

ABDOMINAL AND DIGESTIVE PAIN

Bad abdominal pain can be serious, so expert advice needs to be sought as soon as possible, especially if the pain is so acute it prevents you from standing upright, or if your pain is chronic and you are losing weight, and your stools have become either narrow or dark, or you see blood in them, or if you develop diarrhoea which does not correct itself in a day or so, or if your urine becomes very dark, or you have pain in the upper abdomen and/or you notice a yellow tinge in your skin or in the whites of your eyes.

There are a great many forms of abdominal pain, ranging from appendicitis to gall bladder disease and simple indigestion. Causes can include problems of the large and small intestines, kidneys, stomach, liver, pancreas, ovaries, womb or bladder – and yet for the majority of abdominal pains no obvious cause can be found.

When abdominal pain is chronic (recurs regularly or is more or less constant) an ulcer might be the cause. Gastric ulcers produce pain in an area about the size of a hand placed over the stomach, and commonly comes on soon after starting eating, while duodenal pain is 'smaller', can be pinpointed by one finger, and comes on when no eating has taken place for a while.

When some form of abdominal cancer is the cause of chronic pain a wide range of other symptoms will alert the doctor to this possibility.

Less serious causes are the likeliest, however, including infection which produces diarrhoeas, constipation, gas (which commonly produces colic in children but is frequently the cause of pain in adults too). This last cause may be because poor secretion of digestive enzymes and juices leads to incomplete breakdown of food and consequent fermentation; poor eating habits; smoking; yeast overgrowth (Candida albicans) resulting from antibiotic treatment; intolerance of certain foods such as wheat or milk; or even swallowing air – aerophagia – especially in people who are anxious and who hyperventilate (see section on Chest Pain).

Orthodox medicine
Medical treatment will vary from palliative (antacids) to surgical depending on the causes.

Self-help first-aid

Note: Before applying self-help methods you need to know the cause. It could be fatal to try to take the pain of appendicitis away using self-help measures, thereby leaving it until it burst. If you really know the cause, and are dealing with this responsibly, then there are tactics you can use to obtain relief from pain.

S   The safest and best method of treating most digestive complaints of an acute nature is to fast on apple or carrot juice only for 48 hours.

S   For first-aid treatment (not regular) of constipation use an enema or a suppository, or take two tablespoonsful of linseed (from a Health Food store not a pet food shop!) washed down with lots of water (this provides gel-like bulk), or take Milk of Magnesia.

S   Learn a relaxation method (Autogenic Training) or biofeedback techniques, as these have been shown to help most forms of chronic digestive pain, whether irritable bowel syndrome, colitis or constipation.

S   For relief from haemorrhoid pain use local hot then cold applications (either dunking the area in water of contrasting temperatures, using a small hand shower or applying damp wet cloths of contrasting temperatures – always finishing with cold. Follow with application of petroleum jelly).

S   For rapid easing of itching or burning sensation at the anus (pruritis ani) use neutral (body temperature) sitz bath.

S   For rapid relief from symptoms of bloating, try clay powder (fine French green clay or bentonite). This has the ability to absorb the gas. A teaspoonful of clay stirred into water with a tablespoonful of linseed and then swallowed is the safest way of using it. Alternatively purified charcoal taken after a meal may help in the same way.

S   A cold (warming) compress soothes most abdominal pain after about 20 minutes. Leave in place until dry (up to eight hours).

S   For acute colic pain from gall bladder conditions, if the pain refers to the shoulder blade area, lie on something (tennis ball) which can press that spot – it often eases the pain.

S   For relief from heartburn take lemon juice or cider vinegar in hot water, sipped slowly, or drink slowly one of the following herbal teas: mint, parsley, chamomile, raspberry leaf.

S   If the indigestion is accompanied by a lot of flatulence, drink an infusion of angelica (pour a pint of boiling water onto an ounce/25 grams of the cut root and allow to stand for ten minutes) or chew the leaves or raw root.

Counter-irritation
NS Acupuncture is useful in normalizing some digestive problems.
ES TENS can assist in calming many chronic abdominal pains.

Herbal
S   Aloe vera juice – an ounce or two (25–50 grams) in a tumbler of water taken three times a day has a very soothing influence on the entire digestive tract. It is also anti-fungal and therefore kills yeasts such as Candida.
S   Peppermint (in its various forms) is a superb aid to normalizing recurrent indigestion problems.
S   Ginger root in various forms helps normalize digestion. This seems to absorb excess acid. Two or three capsules of the powdered root after meals helps calm acid problems without side-effects.
S   Inflamed bowels are soothed by pure slippery elm powder taken as a paste with liquid.
S   Charcoal powder stirred into a little olive oil is helpful in treating pain for abdominal distension and flatulence, and even spastic colon pain may be helped by taking eight charcoal tablets three times daily.
S   Swedish bitters (includes golden seal, gentian root and wormwood) taken just before meals helps establish adequate acid secretions when these are low (a common cause of bloating). Low acid levels are found in most people who have allergies (such as eczema and asthma) and acne rosacea.
S   Haemorrhoid pain can be alleviated by pilewort (lesser celandine) or golden seal.

Homoeopathy
S   Carbo veg 6X for indigestion and flatulence.
S   China 3X for indigestion and diarrhoea.
S   Nux vomica 6X for indigestion which follows eating fatty food or which has a burning character to it.

S   Haemorrhoid pain can be alleviated by Hamamelis 3X (if there is also back pain), or Nux vomica 3X.

Hydrotherapy
The following will be useful for all forms of digestive upsets, acute or chronic, including hiatus hernia:

S   Cold (warming) compress to the trunk overnight.
S   Wet sheet pack overnight.
S   Alternating hot and cold compresses or fomentations to the stomach, liver area or spine.
S   Hot water bottle or hot towels over the stomach area after meals.
S   Ice bag over stomach area before meals.
S   For painful haemorrhoids – hot sitz bath. When less inflamed – hot and cold.

Nutrition
S   Most digestive problems are helped by eating slowly, chewing well, avoiding large meals, never combining fruits with vegetables, fruits with starches or liquids with solids, avoiding fried food and very strong spices or very hot or cold foods, not eating when stressed, not eating when you are sick (especially if you have a temperature).

ES   Lack of digestive enzymes or hydrochloric acid in sufficient quantity causes a lot of indigestion. These can be supplemented, although advice from a nutritional expert should be sought before doing so.

NS   Food allergies cause a great deal of digestive disturbance and these should be tracked down by an expert.

ES   Fasting (water or diluted juice only) for 24 to 48 hours is the best way of dealing with most digestive problems, and although this is safe to do unsupervised in most instances, consulting a naturopathic practitioner is a good idea to be sure to understand what to expect when fasting.

NS   Many problems which cause pain, including bloating, gas, irritable bowel and constipation, result from yeast (Candida albicans) overgrowth. This occurs most commonly in people who have a history of antibiotic or steroid use. Yeast problems need to be dealt with by a nutritional expert familiar with such conditions. Use of antifungal substances (garlic, aloe vera, olive oil, caprylic acid from coconuts etc.) plus repopulation of friendly bacteria (acidophilus for the small intestine and bifidobacteria for the colon) are major parts of an anti-yeast programme, along with a very low sugar intake.

S   Apple cider vinegar in water for heartburn pain is a proven folk remedy.

S   Using digestive enzymes (available at Health Food stores) with meals helps digestion of foods and prevents gas build-up from fermentation of partially digested food.

Manipulation and massage

NS If low back muscles are very tight and short this will cause reflex weakening of abdominal muscles and consequent sagging of internal organs. If this occurs in anyone with chronic digestive problems, including constipation, osteopathic or other soft tissue approaches to normalization will be helpful.

NS Hiatus hernia is caused by a bulging of the stomach upwards through the diaphragm. This structure can be weakened and distorted by mechanical forces involving the spine, the lower ribs and certain muscles (*psoas*, *quadratus lumborum*) which merge with it if they are not mechanically normal. Osteopathic and chiropractic approaches can help this underlying cause. Breathing retraining and postural re-education are needed to take recovery further.

NS Skilled massage can help many chronic abdominal problems, especially relating to sagging organs and constipation.

Stress reduction

ES Biofeedback is very useful in helping conditions such as irritable bowel syndrome, various forms of ulceration and constipation.

NS Hypnosis is also useful in treating such conditions, especially if anxiety/stress factors have been features of, or have resulted from, these conditions.

BLADDER, KIDNEY AND PROSTATE PAIN

Orthodox medicine

Cystitis is a common female problem, while prostate conditions are entirely a male problem, but kidney pain (sometimes involving what is said to be the worst pain anyone can suffer – the passing of kidney stones) can affect either sex. Medical attention to these includes use of a variety of antibiotic, hormonal and other drugs, and in the case of prostate disease, sometimes surgical interventions.

Self-help first-aid

S   Start immediately to consume large amounts of liquid.

S   For cystitis, take cranberry extract (capsule or liquid) as this dramatically stops bacteria from 'sticking' to the walls of the bladder, allowing them to be washed away.

For prostate and cystitis/urethritis pain:

S   A hot sitz bath, or . . .

S   . . .for prostate problems hot towels applied over the lower abdomen and between the legs.

For acute kidney stone (colic) pain:

S   A hot bath gives relief, albeit temporary, or . . .

S   . . . hot mustard (a teaspoonful to a gallon of water) footbath (NOT IF DIABETIC) together with a blanket to cover the rest of your body (to maintain warmth) and cold forehead compress, or . . .

S   . . . hot trunk pack, renewed every 10–15 minutes until relief is felt.

Herbal

S   Hot buchu tea. Drink one cup per hour during acute cystitis episodes until acute symptoms calm down.

S   Cranberry treatment for cystitis.

S   Parsley tea or watermelon seed tea for cystitis/urethritis pain.

S   Apple cider vinegar drinks to help dissolve kidney stones and for bladder problems.

S   Garlic capsules, 3–6 daily as a natural antibiotic.
S   Aromatherapy juniper oil massage (three drops of oil to an eggcupful of almond oil) or bath (six drops of oil added to bath).

Homoeopathy
S   If cystitis is accompanied by burning pain: Cantharis 3X.
S   If there is a painful urge to urinate, but little result: Nux vomica 3X.
S   If cystitis resulted from exposure to damp/cold: Dulcemara 3X.

Hydrotherapy
S   See first-aid notes above.
S   Epsom salts compress to trunk for kidney stones.

Nutrition
S   A liquid-only fast for 48 hours is indicated for cystitis/urethritis, drinking mainly 'potassium broth' (and water). Potassium broth is made by boiling a variety of vegetables, including parsley, potato skins and a number of green and root vegetables. After simmering for 15 minutes, allow to stand and cool, then strain off the liquid. This is the broth.
S   There are strategies to help prevent ever suffering from kidney stones, and these include:
S   Drinking copious amounts of water daily.
S   Avoiding tea (high in oxalic acid) and hard water.
S   Eating a high fibre diet. This reduces calcium absorption and thereby the likelihood of stone formation.
S   Supplementing with magnesium (400mg daily) to increase solubility of calcium oxalate, thereby reducing risk of stone formation.
S   Supplementing with vitamin B6 (200mg daily) keeps calcium oxalate in solution, thus preventing stone formation.
S   Taking 3–6g of vitamin C daily.

Manipulation and massage
NS Massage of the prostate can help restore this to normal, along with a programme of hydrotherapy, nutritional changes (zinc and pollen supplementation and the use of specific amino acids) and herbs, such as *Serenoa repens* (saw palmetto) under the direction of a naturopath or herbal practitioner.

GYNAECOLOGICAL (PELVIC) AND MENSTRUAL PAIN

Orthodox medicine

As with other major areas of the body (chest, abdomen) problems affecting this region are diverse, with many possible causes ranging from infectious to hormonal imbalance and growths (benign and malignant). There are also simple structural reasons for some problems.

Sadly, many instances have been reported of unnecessary surgery in cases of pelvic pain syndrome where nothing organically wrong has been discovered, only for the cause to be later identified as trigger point activity. If this were a first line of investigation many instances of unnecessary treatment could be avoided.

Medical treatment of pain in this area will, therefore, depend on just what is going on and what is causing it; and it might include hormonal or antibiotic drugs of various sorts. Many painful conditions relating to infection of sexual origin are possible – chlamydia, herpes and candida being among the most common.

Self-help first-aid

S   Menstrual and vaginal (vaginismus) cramps can be eased by immersion in hot water (tolerable, not scalding) to which has been added bicarbonate of soda or Epsom salts. Stay in the hot bath for up to half-an-hour.

S   Hot sitz bath for these conditions.

Note: Do not use hot immersion if there is haemorrhage. Cold only should be used in such cases. Do not use cold baths for spasm.

S   Exercise (a brisk walk) and deep breathing both relieve menstrual cramp pains for many people.

NS Massage of the low back, if correctly applied, can relieve menstrual cramps rapidly.

S   Self-treatment using acupressure is helpful. Find points which are sensitive about two to three inches directly below the umbilicus. Maintain deep pressure on the sensitive point as you inhale, and lighten pressure as you exhale. Repeat this ten times.

S   If you have backache related to gynaecological (e.g. menstrual) conditions, stuff two tennis balls into the toe of a sock, tie it, and lie on them so that one ball is on each side of your spine at a level which feels sore, but which gives a 'nice' hurt when pressed (usually just below the lower ribs). Maintain for several minutes.

S Drink raspberry leaf tea which has been allowed to stew for several minutes.

S If there is severe discomfort around the vagina because of thrush (yeast) use one of the following methods of relief:

Live yogurt applied to the area (ideally to which you have added several teaspoonsful of powdered acidophilus culture). If the burning itch is internal, use a tampon soaked in the yogurt for a few hours.

Douche with diluted aloe vera juice (1 fl oz to a tumbler of water). Internal use via tampon is also helpful.

Tea tree oil is a powerful antifungal agent, and pessaries are available containing this, or the oil can be applied locally wherever itch/burn exists.

Diluted vinegar can be very soothing for itching and burning.

S As with labour pains, the pains of menstruation can be dramatically eased by deep relaxation and breathing methods which have been practised when pain free. About 20 minutes practise every day, and application for two 20-minute periods daily when pain is present works wonders for many people.

Counter-irritation

ES TENS is very effective in masking period and other pelvic pains.

NS Acupuncture treatment can help chronic pelvic pain, especially if trigger points can be found.

Herbal

ES *Vibernum prunifolium* (black haw): 15–20 drops of tincture in water for menstrual cramps, three times a day as needed.

ES *Viburnum opulus* (cramp bark): 15–20 drops of tincture for uterine cramps, three times a day as needed.

ES Ginger root, eaten, or as an infusion, or in tablet form, for general menstrual pain.

S Garlic relieves heavy painful clotting at period time, and up to six capsules of garlic oil can be taken daily at this time.

S   Caraway oil (six drops in a bath) is helpful as an aromatherapy treatment for painful menstrual conditions.

S   For painful vaginal infections, use oil of sage (six drops in a bath) or local washing of area (three drops in a bidet or basin).

Homoeopathy

S   For cramp-like pains which improve with warmth: Mag phos 3X.

S   If period pain is extreme and feels better for being pressed: Colocynthis 6X.

S   If pain is extreme and you feel very irritable: Chamomilla 3X.

Hydrotherapy

Note: Hydrotherapy measures, such as hot applications to pelvic areas (see above and below) can be started a week before the period is due. Ensure at this time, and throughout the period, that your legs and feet are kept warm.

S   Alternating hot and cold sitz baths twice daily (at each there is a hot-cold alternation twice, i.e. hot-cold-hot-cold) for menstrual pain if not acute spasm, or for pelvic congestion.

S   Ice pack to area overlying uterus and pubis for menstrual pain, 15 minutes per hour.

S   Hot fomentations to lower abdomen for painful periods before flow has started. Repeat every five minutes or so, three times. Give together with hot footbath and cold application to the head, if possible. Wrap warmly afterwards. Repeat two or three times daily until flow begins.

Nutrition

S   The following supplements are known to ease chronic menstrual irregularity and pain:

magnesium (500mg daily);

vitamin B6 (200mg daily);

vitamin E (400 iu daily) – especially if painful breast swelling/ sensitivity occurs with premenstrual build-up;

evening primrose oil (1,500 mg daily).

Manipulation and massage

NS Massage to the low back – deep and slow is very helpful for menstrual pain of all sorts.

NS Osteopathic or chiropractic treatment of low back area is helpful for chronic conditions of menstrual irregularity/pain.

NS Research has shown that many women suffer chronic and acute pelvic pain because of trigger points in the muscles of the inner thigh, the lower abdomen and sometimes even in the muscles of the genitalia. Research has shown that treatment by use of anaesthetic injections (procaine) helped over 90 per cent of one group of over 100 women to achieve freedom from chronic pelvic pain, and to thus avoid exploratory surgical investigation. Many of these triggers can be treated using soft lasers or manual methods (massage and soft tissue manipulation).

Stress reduction methods

ES Biofeedback is of major importance in helping people with chronic pelvic and menstrual pain to achieve improved control of their pain.

NS Hypnosis can achieve similar relief.

S Deep relaxation, involving methods of breathing and Autogenic Training-type relaxation, allows improved circulation and muscle tone to be developed.

CHILDBIRTH

Counter-irritation
NS A skilled acupuncturist can help relieve the pains of childbirth.

Herbal
S Raspberry leaf tea before and during labour.

Homoeopathy
S To encourage easy delivery: Caulophyllum 6X.

S To ease false pains: Gelsemium 3X.

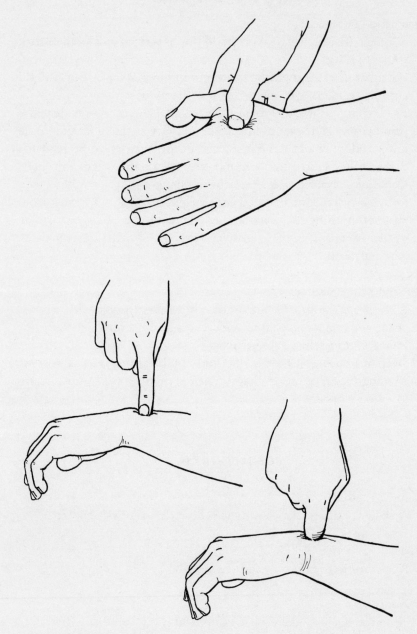

FIGURE 44 The thumbs, finger tips or knuckles can be used to apply acupressure to muscles and/or trigger points.

Hydrotherapy

NS Underwater birth is claimed to make delivery far easier and more 'natural'. This is only to be attempted under expert supervision.

S Long neutral or warm baths are helpful in easing late pregnancy discomfort.

Manipulation and massage

ES Massage to the low back has a remarkable effect on pain levels during labour.

ES Acupressure (Shiatsu) methods of applying pressure to specific areas can relieve the discomfort and pain of childbirth:

> Firm pressure on a point found the width of the person's hand above the ankle, on the inner aspect of either leg;
>
> Pain in the back is relieved by firm pressure just below the last rib near the spine;
>
> Pain is eased if tender points on the sacrum (very lowest part of the spine just above the coccyx) are firmly pressed.

NS Osteopathic attention before delivery (ideally for the last three months of pregnancy), at monthly intervals, can help prepare bony structure (pelvic bones mainly) for delivery and can ease discomfort of late pregnancy.

Stress-reduction

S Breathing exercises are an essential method for achieving control over the discomfort of childbirth and for preparing for it without anxiety.

S Deep relaxation methods are helpful in releasing muscular tensions which develop as pregnancy advances.

VARICOSE VEINS

Orthodox medicine

Once veins lose their efficiency (valves break down and allow a back-flow of blood causing veins to swell) it is almost impossible to restore normality. The best that can be done is to avoid aggravating them, and to provide relief from the symptoms of heavy aching (wear support tights, avoid prolonged standing, rest legs on a footstool when sitting etc). Medically, surgery or blocking the affected vein by injection are the ultimate answers – which then leaves the remaining veins to cope with the additional load previously carried by the now absent or blocked vein or veins. If a thrombosis is threatening, a blood-thinning drug may be used.

Self-help first-aid

S   Stop smoking if you are a smoker, and lose weight if you are overweight.

S   Take the load off your feet, and avoid standing wherever possible. Sit with feet higher than hips. Wear support tights if you do have to stand a lot, and keep moving.

S   Remove or loosen anything tight around the waist, whether this is a belt, corset or other clothing. Similarly, remove anything tight around the leg such as elasticated knee-high sock support or tight panties.

S   When veins/legs are aching and painful, apply warm or hot towels to the area for five minutes at a time, several times, and then finish with a cold application (30 seconds).

S   Cold spraying your legs with a hand-held shower helps reduce congestion.

Homoeopathy

S   Pulsatilla 3X or Hamamelis 3X.

S   If veins are inflamed (phlebitis): Vipera 3X.

ES If vein is bleeding (without obvious injury to it): Hamamelis 3X should be taken every 20 minutes. A doctor should be called. Meanwhile, you should lie down with your leg elevated as high as possible, and the area above and below the bleeding vein should be bandaged.

Herbal

S   Use of lemon oil is helpful if massaged locally over the vein area, or put six drops in a warm bath (always follow a bath with a cold shower to your legs).

Hydrotherapy

S   Daily hot and cold sitz baths, morning and evening to help pelvic congestion/circulation.

S   Local application (30 minutes twice daily if possible) over veins of compress soaked in tepid water, to which has been added calendula oil or witch hazel.

S   Local hot and cold applications (towel rung out in water of appropriate temperature) over veins. Three minutes hot and 30 seconds cold, repeated four or five times, and always finishing with cold.

Nutrition

S   Avoiding constipation is important, as any increase in abdominal pressure increases back-pressure to the veins, making matters worse. Adding a fibre (linseed, for example) to the diet can deal with this.

S   Supplementation with bioflavonoids and vitamin C (3g daily); vitamin E (400 iu daily) and a daily multi-mineral supplement is helpful.

S   Rutin (extract of buckwheat) is a useful bioflavonoid for helping veins. This is available as a tablet or as a dried herb which can be taken as a tea.

S   If it is suggested that there may be a thrombosis in the vein (a clot partially blocking its course) then take as much garlic as you can (raw or in capsule form – six to eight daily) as well as 600 iu of vitamin E daily and 3g of vitamin C, along with whatever the doctor is giving for the problem. Inform your doctor of what you are doing.

Stress reduction

S   Yoga postures, such as shoulder stand or others in which the body is inverted, help circulation, especially if breathing exercises accompany these.

S   Breathing produces a pumping action which helps venous circulation, and slow deep breathing using the diaphragm is essential to reduce back-pressure to the legs.

S   Walking is the best exercise of all, so that muscles can alternately contract and relax, producing a muscle pump action which helps the veins move stagnant blood.

SKIN DISEASES

Self-help first-aid
See Herbal and Hydrotherapy sections below.

Counter-irritation
NS Acupuncture combined with the use of traditional Chinese herbs has proved helpful in chronic skin problems such as eczema.
ES TENS applied across a painful skin lesion will reduce the intensity of what is being felt.

Healing/Therapeutic Touch
NS Chronic problems in particular respond well to healing methods.

Herbal
NS If there are low levels of hydrochloric acid secretions in the stomach, contributing to allergic reactions (see Nutrition below), then use of Swedish bitters (a combination of herbs) can improve digestive function.
S Extract of witch hazel, or marigold, or chickweed diluted in water and applied to the painful area as a compress (tepid not hot) soothes most local skin conditions.
S For facial herpes or dry eczema add three drops of geranium oil to a little (eggcupful) almond oil and apply three times daily.
S For dry eczema, oil of hyssop mixed with an eggcupful almond oil can be applied daily.
S For wet eczema four drops of juniper oil to an eggcupful of almond oil can be applied to the areas affected twice daily.
S A most useful application to the skin for any condition (burns, shingles, fungal infections, stings, infected wounds etc.) is aloe vera, either as diluted or neat juice, or as a gel, or the sap directly from the plant if this is available.
S For raw chapped skin use calendula ointment.

Homoeopathy
S Herpes: Natrum mur 3X or 6X.
S For herpes or eczema: Rhus tox 3X.

S   For urticaria (hives): Apis mellifica 3X or Urtica urens 3X.

Hydrotherapy

NS   Under supervision only (health resort ideally) an oxygen (peroxide) bath helps most skin problems dramatically. A hot bath has added to it a tablespoonful of potassium permanganate, 1½ tablespoonsful sulphuric acid and 12 oz (300g) hydrogen peroxide. The water will bubble, and 20 minutes resting in the bath, followed by patting skin dry and resting, helps ease pain of most dermatitis conditions.

S   To relieve skin irritation from most causes, 20–30 minutes in a warm alkaline (not very hot) bath containing bicarbonate of soda (one cupful) is useful (urticaria, eczema, shingles pain, heat rash, allergic reactions to chemicals or plants, insect stings, sunburn etc.).

S   For these same conditions an oatmeal bath can be used. The water should be fairly warm, but not very hot. Add a few tablespoonsful of finely ground uncooked oatmeal powder to the bath, and tie into a cloth at least 1 lb (450g) of coarse uncooked oatmeal. Hang this from the tap so that the water runs through it. When the bath is full, remove this and use it as a sponge to gently pat areas of particular irritation. Half-an-hour in the oatmeal bath, followed by patting the skin dry, is indicated daily.

ES   For psoriasis spend 45 minutes every day in a neutral bath with 1 lb (450g) or more of sea salt dissolved in it. Pat dry afterwards.

Nutrition

ES   Most acute and chronic skin conditions are helped by controlled fasting (never more than 48 hours without supervision). Fasting is best done at a health resort where help is at hand, since the condition can get worse for a few days before improving.

ES   For skin health adequate intake of vitamin A (if supplementing take beta-carotene), zinc, vitamins B and C.

ES   Many skin conditions are of allergic origin (urticaria, eczema etc.) and so a diet needs to be constructed which avoids the particular substances/foods which provoke the condition. A skilled nutritional expert is needed for this.

NS   Hydrochloric acid secretions are often deficient in people with such skin conditions, and supplementation with this in capsule form may help (see Herbal above).

ES For recurrent herpes simplex (cold sores or genital herpes) a diet low in arginine-rich foods and high in lysine-rich foods is suggested. Advice from a nutrition counsellor or naturopath is indicated. Take 1–1½g lysine (an amino acid) daily, away from meals as this retards herpes virus activity.

Stress reduction

S Stress reduction through breathing, relaxation and meditation exercises has a beneficial effect on all chronic skin diseases, just as stress has a negative effect on them.

ES Biofeedback has been shown in research studies to lead to reduction in intensity of many inflammatory skin problems.

NS Hypnosis is also of proven value in dealing with many painful or irritating skin problems.

ABSCESSES, BOILS AND SKIN ULCERS

Herbal

S Granulated sugar or honey applied to open wounds/ulcers speeds healing and soothes pain.

S Apply thyme oil (three drops to a cup of warm water) to the area of a boil or septic wound, using cotton wool, to soothe and promote healing.

S Bruise cabbage leaves or finely grate them and apply as a poultice (wrapped in gauze) over the boil whether it is open or not yet open. Replace daily until it is healed.

Hydrotherapy

S For abscesses apply hot and cold towels. The water should have had Epsom salts dissolved in it (half a cupful to a basin of water). Repetitions of two minutes hot, one minute cold should continue for eight to ten times, two or three times daily.

S If the abscess is on the legs or the trunk then soak in an Epsom salts bath to help it to draw.

Nutrition

ES Nutritional approaches to boils and abscesses and wound healing demand a raw food diet for up to a week (fruit and salads only, plus ample liquid, and/or water only fast, 48 hours). Expert advice from a naturopathic practitioner or a nutrition counsellor should be sought for advice on the best way to apply these.

Supplements: Vitamin B complex, vitamin A, vitamin C and bioflavanoids.

CHILBLAINS AND FROSTBITE

Self-help first-aid
Frostbite is a serious condition and requires emergency care.

S While waiting for this to arrive apply to the affected area:
     Cold mashed raw potato (to which salt has been added) or peeled raw cucumber, mashed.

S Take homoeopathic Agaricus muscarius 12X.

S Rub the affected area with snow, and then apply cold water while rubbing, and later apply just barely warm water or rub the area with an alcohol (brandy for example). Never try to warm the area too quickly by placing it near a heat source.

Herbal
S Apply tincture of myrrh and massage . . .

S . . . or rub in Friar's balsam.

Homoeopathy
S If the condition is worse when you are hot: Pulsatilla 6X.

S If swollen and worse when hot: Apis mellifica.

Hydrotherapy
S For chilblains, place hands or feet in hot water for two minutes, then immediately plunge into cold water for one minute. Repeat five more times, finishing with cold. Do this twice daily.

S   For non-bleeding chilblains a compress wrung out in cold water, into which arnica tincture has been placed (six drops to a pint of water) can be applied to the painful area and left on overnight.

S   If the area is bleeding, then apply calendula cream after the hot and cold alternations described above.

Nutrition

S   For frostbite take one high-potency vitamin B-complex capsule, and 400 iu vitamin E daily.

S   For chilblains: 3g vitamin C, 1g bioflavonoids, 400 iu vitamin E daily, and a multi-mineral tablet.

CRAMP

Cramp occurs when, for one reason or another, not enough circulation gets to a particular area, and the muscle, starved of oxygen, goes into spasm.

Self-help first-aid

S   Try to stretch the muscle (for example, if it is in the calf muscle, by standing and leaning forward with foot flat on the floor) or . . .

S   . . . find the 'centre' of the pain and press in deeply with thumb(s) while gently trying to stretch the area.

S   Apply a hot wet towel to the area after the cramp has eased, or while it is still easing. Repeat every five minutes four or five times, and then move the muscle gently, by walking or stretching.

S   Massage upwards towards the heart, squeezing and kneading the muscle.

Herbal

S   Cramp bark (as an infusion) or kelp taken as powder (in capsule or tablet form).

Homoeopathy

S   Cuprum metallicum 3X.

Hydrotherapy

S   Hot (1–2 minutes) and cold (15–30 seconds) applications (wet towels or hand shower application) to the area when cramp is absent.

Nutrition

S   Evening primrose oil: 1,000mg daily.

S   Vitamins C (3g daily) and E (400 iu daily) are useful.

S   Deficiency of sodium (as in salt) and magnesium are both causes of cramp in muscles. Ensure adequate salt intake if in a hot climate where sweating is heavy, and of magnesium by supplementing with 500mg daily with food.

Manipulation and massage

S   See Self-help first-aid above.

NS Massage of the body, especially of the limbs if this is where cramp if felt, is a useful long-term strategy.

Folklore

If you tend to suffer from cramp during the night, you might like to try placing a cork under your mattress; this piece of folk medicine is inexplicable but works for many people.

STINGS AND BITES

Self-help first-aid

If stung by a bee, remove the sting with tweezers, or ease it out using a flat needle against the skin.

S   Apply cold running water for up to ten minutes.

S   If stung by a wasp there is no sting to remove. Apply vinegar or lemon juice, or a paste made of bicarbonate of soda, as soon as possible to neutralize the venom.

Caution: If the person stung feels unwell or has difficulty in breathing, he or she may be suffering an acute allergic response to the sting. Get emergency care immediately.

S   For both bee and wasp stings take Ledum homoeopathically (especially if the area feels cold and the symptoms are improved by cold). This is ideal for sharp pricking pains.

S   The pulped heads and buds of young marigolds (calendula) make an excellent tincture (preserved in alcohol) which can be applied to stings and other surface injuries. Or, a pulped fresh flower can be applied directly to a sting and bandaged in place.

Homoeopathy

S   If the area is swollen and shiny take Apis mellifica 6X.

S   For heavy itching around the sting take Urtica 6X.

BURNS AND SCALDS

Remove the source of the burn. Remove any jewellery and clothing in the area of the burn or scald. If the area affected is no bigger than an inch square (3cm across) treat it yourself. If larger, get expert advice and help. If the burn is electrical, get emergency attention.

Caution: Do not apply butter, oil or grease, or burst any blister or cover with cloth which might adhere to the surface. Use gauze bandaging only, and very lightly until expert help is available.

Self-help first-aid

S   Get the area under cold running water and keep it there for as long as you can, but for at least ten minutes (an hour is not too much!) or until help arrives.

S   If the cause is a chemical, then wash with running water after removing any clothing from the area. At least ten minutes of water application is needed.

S   For sunburn apply cold wet packs until irritation subsides, and then use calendula ointment.

Herbal

S   When healing is under way apply diluted lavender oil (four drops in an eggcupful of almond oil).

S   Apply diluted witch hazel soaked gauze and gently bandage the site of small burns and scalds. This stops infection and promotes healing.

S   Aloe vera juice, or the sap of the leaf, or a gel containing it are all soothing and promote healing.

S   Calendula ointment is soothing as healing advances.

Homoeopathy

S   For pain take Cantharis 3X every hour until relief is noted.

S   For severe pain from burns or scalds: Aconitum 12X (one dose only).

S   Dress minor burns and scalds with gauze soaked in mother tincture of Urtica urens (eight drops to half a cup of water).

Hydrotherapy

S   See Self-help first-aid above.

S   A neutral bath maintained for as long as possible is extremely soothing to burn patients (a case is recorded of ten days in a neutral bath, coming out only for toilet needs and for a daily anointing of skin with petrolatum to protect it). Have a cushion for the head. If necessary (for comfort) also have foam on the base of the bath to lie on, and keep feet out of the water to avoid swelling and wrinkling of skin. Water temperature must remain at body temperature throughout.

Nutrition

S   Repair of damage requires large amounts of specific nutrients which can be supplied as supplements. The main ones are vitamin C (3g daily, or more in severe cases) and zinc (50mg daily).

GENERAL/WHOLE BODY PAIN

There are many reasons why some people are obliged to face chronic or periodic whole body pain, including arthritic conditions, a particular blood disease (such as sickle cell anaemia), cancer or infection (such as active herpes zoster or shingles). In a lot of cases the best that medical science has to offer are various forms of pain-killing medication, and while sometimes these are barely adequate, in many instances they are able to control quite high levels of pain.

Research has shown that when there is severe and chronic pain (as in some cases of cancer) the best method of control is the use of narcotic drugs, and that only in a very small percentage does this lead to addiction (six out of 100 people in one study, and all six had severe psychological problems before this medication). The message, then, is that we should not feel that appropriate use of narcotics, in skilled medical hands, is dangerous. In fact, the pain itself can be more destructive until you find a way of controlling it.

And, of course, there are other methods which can be added to such approaches, or which can sometimes replace them. Indeed, all or any of the many methods which have been outlined in this book can also be used to good effect, if available. For example, a full sheet pack or neutral bath can offer very marked pain relief, as can acupuncture, TENS, massage (even if only temporarily), hypnosis, stress-reduction/relaxation methods, nutritional strategies which lower inflammatory substances, various safe herbal compounds and extracts as well as homoeopathic methods. All can work individually and sometimes several of these in concert can offer help.

None of them will always be effective, and trial and error is sometimes necessary to find out which one, or which combination, helps most in a given case. If you remember the basic rules of hydrotherapy, as explained, and use the various combinations, as outlined, of hot and cold, cold (or ice) alone, heat alone or neutral alone, a number of choices are opened up, and many of these can produce great pain relief in very severe conditions, especially when used systematically and regularly.

Massage has been shown to have profound pain relieving effects on chronic pain, although sometimes relief lasts for only a few hours or days. Nevertheless, it is worth repeating for the long-term reduction of stress, anxiety and pain which a sense of being even slightly 'in control' can bring. TENS and acupuncture are also remarkably effective, as are the various deep relaxation methods, including biofeedback and hypnosis.

If you can achieve partial relief from even a part of the pain which had previously been constant and widespread, you are moving forward towards control of it. Chances are that investigation and use of the many choices available in the menu of pain relief methods will help to achieve more than just partial relief . . .and the only way to find out is to discover what works for you by trying what appeals to you most, or what is most readily available.

In the end, pain is in our nervous system, our brains and minds, and whatever else we do we need to come to terms with it and not allow it to dominate our lives. I hope the choices I have listed and the options that are available help you towards an easing, a control and ideally an elimination of your pain.

Bibliography

Bradley, Dinah, *Hyperventilation Syndrome*, Century Arrow 1992
Brennan, Richard, *Alexander Technique Workbook*, Element 1992
Chaitow, Leon, *Clear Body, Clear Mind*, Unwin/Thorsons 1990
—, *Osteopathic Self-Treatment*, Thorsons 1990
—, *Stress Protection Plan*, Thorsons 1992
Cowmeadow, Oliver, *The Art of Shiatsu*, Element 1992
Davies, Stephen and Alan Stewart, *Nutritional Medicine*, Pan Books 1989
King, Robert, *Performance Massage*, Human Kinetics 1992
Macrae, Janet, *Therapeutic Touch*, Knopf 1988
Melzack and Wall, *The Challenge of Pain*, Penguin 1983
Newman Turner, Rodger, *Naturopathic medicine*, Thorsons 1990
Sherwood, Paul, *The Back and Beyond*, Arrow 1992
Trattler, Ross, *Better Health Through Natural Healing*, Thorsons 1985

Index